CONTINUOUS AMBULATORY PERITONEAL DIALYSIS

Other titles in the *New Clinical Applications* Series:

Dermatology (Series Editor Dr J. L. Verbov)
Dermatological Surgery
Superficial Fungal Infections
Talking Points in Dermatology – I
Treatment in Dermatology
Current Concepts in Contact Dermatitis
Talking Points in Dermatology – II
Tumours, Lymphomas and Selected Paraproteinaemias

Cardiology (Series Editor Dr D. Longmore)
Cardiology Screening

Rheumatology (Series Editors Dr J. J. Calabra and Dr W. Carson Dick)
Ankylosing Spondylitis
Infections and Arthritis

Nephrology (Series Editor Professor G. R. D. Catto)
Continuous Ambulatory Peritoneal Dialysis
Management of Renal Hypertension
Chronic Renal Failure
Calculus Disease
Pregnancy and Renal Disorders
Multisystem Diseases
Glomerulonephritis I
Glomerulonephritis II

NEW
CLINICAL
APPLICATIONS
NEPHROLOGY

CONTINUOUS AMBULATORY PERITONEAL DIALYSIS

Editor

G. R. D. CATTO
DSc, MD, FRCP (Lond., Edin. and Glasg.)

Professor in Medicine and Therapeutics
University of Aberdeen
UK

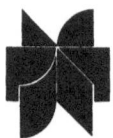

KLUWER ACADEMIC PUBLISHERS
DORDRECHT / BOSTON / LONDON

Distributors

for the United States and Canada: Kluwer Academic Publishers, PO Box 358, Accord Station, Hingham, MA 02018-0358, USA
for all other countries: Kluwer Academic Publishers Group, Distribution Center, PO Box 322, 3300 AH Dordrecht, The Netherlands

British Library Cataloguing in Publication Data

Continuous ambulatory peritoneal dialysis.
1. Ambulatory patients. Kidneys.
Continuous peritoneal dialysis
I. Catto, Graeme R.D. (Graeme Robert
Dawson). *1945–*   II. Series
617'.461059

ISBN-13: 978-94-011-7830-3   e-ISBN-13: 978-94-011-7828-0
DOI: 10.1007/978-94-011-7828-0

Library of Congress Cataloging-in-Publication Data

Continuous ambulatory peritoneal dialysis/editor, G.R.D. Catto.
       p.   cm.——(New clinical applications. Nephrology)
    Includes bibliographies and index.
    ISBN-13: 978-94-011-7830-3
    1. Continuous ambulatory peritoneal dialysis. I. Catto, Graeme
R. D.   II. Series.
    [DNLM: 1. Peritoneal Dialysis, Continuous Ambulatory. WJ 378 C759]
RC901.7.P48C67 1988
617'.461059——dc 19
DNLM/DLC
for Library of Congress   88-23155
                                                                    CIP

Published in the United Kingdom by Kluwer Academic Publishers,
PO Box 55, Lancaster, UK.

Kluwer Academic Publishers BV incorporates the publishing programmes of
D. Reidel, Martinus Nijhoff, Dr W. Junk and MTP Press.

Butler & Tanner Ltd, Frome and London

CONTENTS

LIST OF AUTHORS

R. A. Baillod
Department of Nephrology and
Transp
The Royal Free Hospital
Pond Street,
Hampstead
London, NW3 2QG
UK

A. J. Bint
Department of Microbiology
The Royal Victoria Infirmary
Queen Victoria Road
Newcastle-upon-Tyne, NE1 4LP
UK

C. T. Flynn
1215 Pleasant, Suite 100
Des Moines
Iowa 50309
USA

R. Gokal
Department of Renal Medicine
Manchester Royal Infirmary
Oxford Road
Manchester, M13 9WL
UK

A. J. Nicholls
Kidney Unit
Royal Devon and Exeter
Hospital (Wonford)
Barrack Road
Exeter, Devon EX2 5DW
UK

S. J. Pedler
Department of Microbiology
The Royal Victoria Infirmary
Queen Victoria Road
Newcastle-upon-Tyne, NE1 4LP
UK

SERIES EDITOR'S FOREWORD

For more than a generation haemodialysis has been the principal method of treating patients with both acute and chronic renal failure. Initially, developments and improvements in the system were highly technical and relevant to only a relatively small number of specialists in nephrology. More recently, as advances in therapy have demonstrated the value of haemofiltration in the intensive therapy unit and haemoperfusion for certain types of poisoning, the basic principles of haemodialysis have been perceived as important in many areas of clinical practice.

In this volume, the potential advantages of bicarbonate haemodialysis are objectively assessed, the technical and clinical aspects of both haemofiltration and haemoperfusion discussed and the continuing problems associated with such extra corporeal circuits analysed. All the chapters have been written by recognized experts in their field. The increasing availability of highly technical facilities for appropriately selected patients should ensure that the information contained in the book is relevant not only to nephrologists but to all practising clinicians.

ABOUT THE EDITOR

Dr Graeme R. D. Catto is Professor in Medicine and Therapeutics at the University of Aberdeen and Honorary Consultant Physician/Nephrologist to the Grampian Health Board. His current interest in transplant immunology was stimulated as a Harkness Fellow at Harvard Medical School and the Peter Bent Brighton Hospital, Boston, USA. He is a member of many medical societies including the Association of Physicians of Great Britain and Ireland, the Renal Association and the Transplantation Society. He has published widely on transplant and reproductive immunology, calcium metabolism and general nephrology.

1
CONTINUOUS AMBULATORY PERITONEAL DIALYSIS

R. GOKAL

Although the concept of peritoneal dialysis had been with us for many decades, its use in the management of patients in end stage renal failure was of a limited nature until the introduction of continuous ambulatory peritoneal dialysis (CAPD) in 1976[1]. Since then, interest in peritoneal dialysis has increased tremendously and CAPD has now become an established form of renal replacement therapy, challenging haemodialysis as the first choice dialysis treatment. The current state of the art has been a combination of painstaking efforts on the part of several innovative pioneers in this field[2]. This review outlines the more recent advances in the technique of CAPD and in the understanding of its pathophysiological processes and attempts to correlate these with the results and use of CAPD in chronic renal failure.

PERITONEAL MORPHOLOGY AND PHYSIOLOGY

The CAPD technique, as initially proposed by Popovich and Moncrief[1], entailed four daily exchanges of 2-litre volumes to produce a 10 L dialysate over a 24 hour period. This necessitated 4–8 hour dwell periods adjusted to fit into the patients daily routine. Whereas this concept, based on sound anatomical and physiological considerations, has not changed in the last 10 years and remains the cornerstone of CAPD, the more recent advances in the knowledge of the effect on the peritoneum of peritonitis, the constant presence of dialysis fluid in the peritoneal cavity and subsequent changes of solute and fluid removal have had a major impact on CAPD.

The peritoneal membrane consists of three layers, the capillary endothelium, the peritoneal interstitium and the mesothelial layer containing many cytoplasmic vesicles with projecting microvilli (Figure 1.1). Entrapped within this layer of microvilli is a thin layer of fluid containing a surface acting material, phosphotidylcholine (a surfactant), which not only acts as a surface lubricant but prevents further damage to the mesothelium; it may also be important in maintaining ultrafiltration[3]. The mesothelial layer is held together by desmosomes and tight junctions. The interstitium contains fibroblasts, mast cells, elastic tissue and bundles of collagen[4]. The introduction of peritoneal dialysis fluid into this membrane cavity has profound ultrastructural effects. These include the development of mesothelial intracellular oedema, disruption of organelles, interstitial oedema and

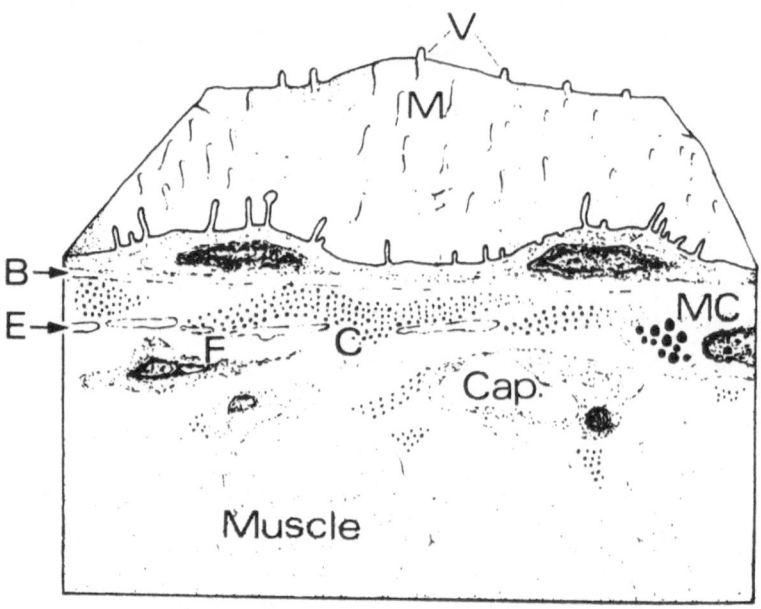

FIGURE 1.1   Normal appearance of the peritoneal membrane showing the mesothelial cell layer (M) with abundant microvilli (V). Granulated mast cells (MC) and fibroblasts (F) are identified as are basement membrane (B), elastic tissue (E) and collagen (C). (Reproduced with permission, Churchill Livingstone)

submesothelial deposition of collagen fibres[4,5]. After several months of CAPD the distance between the mesothelial surface and the capillaries increases to 20–40 μm[4].

Solute transfer

The transfer of solutes and fluid across the peritoneal membrane is opposed by at least six major 'resistances' to diffusion, mainly the stagnant fluid films adjacent to the capillary endothelium and the mesothelium[6]. The structural changes found after peritoneal dialysis may also influence the solute and water kinetics. The nature of this passage depends on the physicochemical properties of the individual substances – neutral non-colloidal substances, e.g. urea, will pass by passive *diffusion*. In addition, the flux of fluid across the peritoneum in response to osmotic agents induces the movement of solutes in the absence of a concentration gradient; thus solute transport occurs partly by *convection* or 'solvent drag'[7].

Peritoneal dialysis relies on the transport of metabolites and fluid in the appropriate quantities to maintain the patient in fluid and electrolyte balance. Several mathematical models have been defined to describe these transport phenomena. Whatever the model, peritoneal clearance is a complex function of blood flow, peritoneal dialysis flow rate and the mass transfer area coefficient (a measure of the ability of metabolites to transfer across the peritoneum, a concept that takes into account the area of the peritoneal membrane and the precise 'pore area' available for mass transfer; both of these are, however, difficult to ascertain).

The two theories that encompass these phenomena and are utilized to give a mathematical evaluation of solute transport are the homogeneous (or membrane) theory[8] and Dedrick's distributed theory[9]. The former utilizes a two compartment model with a simple exponential decay of concentration gradient between body fluids and dialysate. Popovich and colleagues expanded this model to include the effects of metabolite generation, protein binding and non-equilibrium distribution[10]. To account for the convection element of solute transport, the relationship between solute and membrane 'pore size' (the reflection coefficient) was incorporated into the mathematical model.

3

Using this, Moncrief and Popovich theorized that a patient will maintain a steady blood urea level of about 30 mmol/L if 10 L of peritoneal dialysis fluid is allowed to equilibrate with body fluids (2 L × 4; dwell time 5–6 hours, 2 L ultrafiltrate). The other theory by Dedrick uses a distributed model of solute transport which visualizes most structures into which peritoneal transport occurs as distributed capillary beds covered by a thin anatomic membrane.

Changes in mass transfer coefficients with time on CAPD have been variably reported but by and large are maintained for up to two to four years[11]. As patients are now maintained for longer periods on CAPD the evaluation of solute transfer parameters will be of paramount importance.

Ultrafiltration

The removal of excess fluid is a critical factor in any form of dialysis; in CAPD this has traditionally been achieved by adding to the solution various concentrations of dextrose, which acts as an osmotic agent. Until recently the view has been that ultrafiltration continues until the dialysate becomes virtually isotonic, after which a gradual fall in intra-abdominal volume occurs as fluid is reabsorbed through the action of plasma oncotic pressure. The intraperitoneal dialysate volume increases rapidly over the first two hours before declining and this phenomenon can be studied by using various markers including labelled albumin, dextran or autologous haemoglobin[12]. Recent work, however, challenges this simplistic view.

During peritoneal dialysis, water may transfer across the peritoneal capillaries in either direction depending on hydrostatic, oncotic and crystalloid osmotic pressures between blood to interstitium and interstitium to peritoneal cavity. Hitherto, the role of lymphatic absorption has been largely disregarded. The major area of peritoneal fluid absorption is the diaphragmatic lymphatics which lie immediately beneath the peritoneum and run parallel with the muscle fibres. When large size particles are introduced into the peritoneal cavity they are readily absorbed by lymphatics, all of which have numerous terminal channels or lacunae which anastamose freely with each other and are localized beneath the mesothelial covering of the peritoneal surface of

4

the diaphragm[23]. The lacunae consist of a sheet of mesothelial cells, a layer of connective tissue and an inner layer of endothelium. The lacunae are situated between radial bundles of collagen fibres. The rate of absorption from the peritoneal cavity depends upon diaphragmatic movements especially during respiration. The diaphragm relaxes in expiration causing the lacunae to dilate; during inspiration the lacunae are compressed and the lymph is expelled into connecting lymph vessels[23]. The material is prevented from being expelled back into the peritoneal cavity by the presence of an overlapping endothelium covering many of the openings of the lacunae[24].

The transcapillary ultrafiltration rate is maximal at the onset of the exchange and decreases exponentially as the crystalloid osmotic pressure declines. The intraperitoneal volume increases until it reaches a maximum when the rate of transcapillary transport equals the rate of peritoneal lymphatic absorption plus that which transfers across the peritoneal capillaries. Net reabsorption begins when lymphatic absorption rate exceeds the transcapillary ultrafiltration rate and continues after crystalloid osmotic equilibrium (Figure 1.2). Osmotic equilibrium is reached before glucose equilibrium since there is a sieving (converse of reflection coefficient) of small solutes with ultrafiltration yet reabsorption via the lymphatics continues (Figure 1.2). Lymphatic reabsorption thus plays an important role in ultrafiltration in peritoneal dialysis.

Shear *et al.*[14] reported the absorption of 0.9% saline from the peritoneal cavity of renal failure patients at a steady rate of 30–37 ml/h whilst a similar study by Daugirdas *et al.* gave values of 26–131 ml/h[15]. The mean lymphatic flow rate determined by the rate of transfer of RISA in 10 CAPD patients was 11.1 ml/h[16]. Factors that diminish lymphatic absorption are upright posture and small intraperitoneal volumes[17]. More recently, some startling results have been reported by Mactier *et al.*[18] who calculated that cumulative lymphatic drainage in the supine position over four hours in CAPD patients ranged from 45–76% of total transcapillary ultrafiltration using 2L of 2.25% dextrose solutions. Whereas this may be a somewhat exaggerated figure because of the supine posture it illustrates the important role of the diaphragmatic lymphatics and may explain why some patients *de novo* have poor ultrafiltration at the start of CAPD. Fluid is also reabsorbed across the peritoneal membrane based on the oncotic

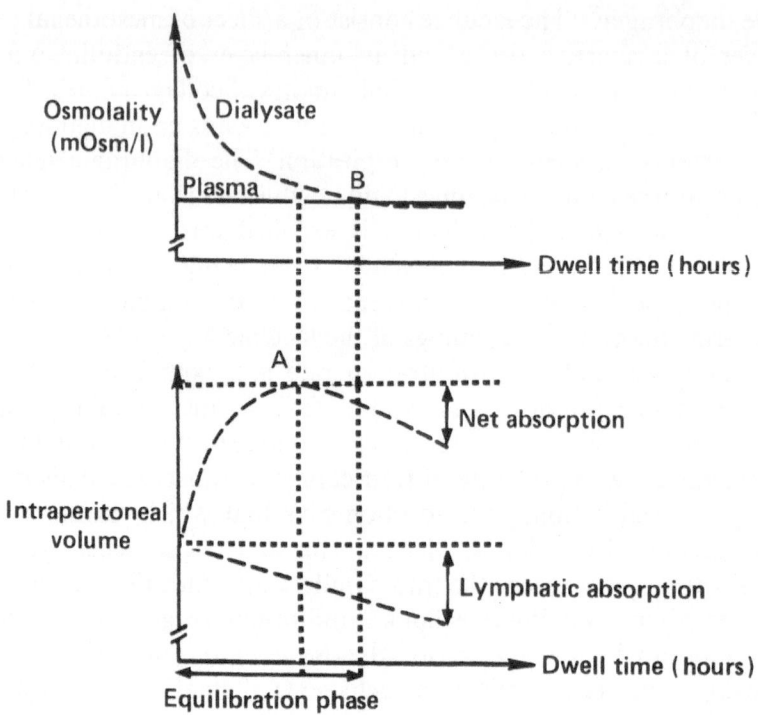

FIGURE 1.2 Diagrammatic representation of ultrafiltration, intra-peritoneal volume and lymphatic reabsorption in a CAPD patient with glucose dialysis. Peak intraperitoneal volume is represented by point A which precedes crystalloid osmotic equilibrium (point B). Volume of net absorption represents the sum of both lymphatic and transcapillary loss. At peak ultrafiltration, lymphatic absorption rate equals transcapillary ultrafiltration rate. (Reproduced with permission of R. Khanna)

pressure in the plasma relative to that in the dialysate. The relative importance of these two processes on the final resultant ultrafiltration has not, however, been determined.

Osmotic agents

Although glucose is relatively cheap and safe, its absorption leads to short lived ultrafiltration and metabolic complications[20], whilst the hyperosmolar nature of the fluid may be deleterious to the membrane and macrophages. Alternative osmotic agents (amino acids, dextrans, gelatin) with less transcapillary absorption than glucose have been sought to induce more effective ultrafiltration in peritoneal dialysis[19,20]. Although macromolecules have minimal transcapillary uptake, transport via the lymphatics means that these will still be absorbed, albeit more slowly.

One such macromolecule of major interest is glucose polymer, isolated by fractionation of hydrolysed corn starch. Mistry *et al.*[21] showed sustained ultrafiltration over 12 hours using a preparation of mol. wt. 20 000 containing dextrins of chain length in excess of 12 glucose units, in spite of the solution being isosmotic to plasma (Figure 1.3). The concept of osmotic water flow in the apparent absence of an osmotic gradient may appear confusing as ultrafiltration is thought

GLUCOSE POLYMER (20,000)

Dialysate osmolality Mean + SEM (n=5)

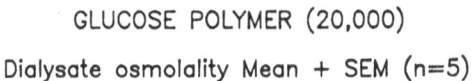

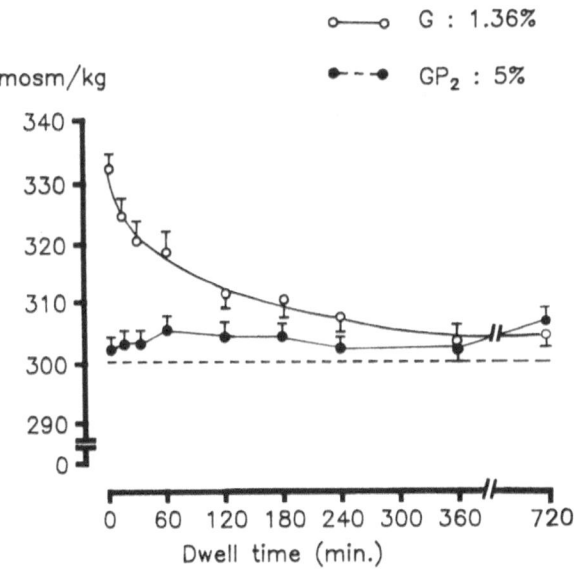

FIGURE 1.3 Dialysate osmolality using glucose polymer solution (mol. wt. 20 000) as compared to 1.36% glucose over a 12 h dwell

7

to be the difference in total osmolality between dialysate and serum. Two important factors contribute to this; the permeable nature of the peritoneal membrane and the large size of the glucose polymer.

Whereas the osmotic flow rate through a semipermeable membrane is primarily dependent on the total number of solute particles, the flow through a permeable membrane is only a function of the number of large, relatively impermeable solutes and unrelated to the total osmolality. Since the variable membrane permeability of solute is characterized by the reflection coefficient, whose value may range from zero (for molecules as permeable as water) to unity (for one that is completely impermeable), the magnitude of the osmotic flow is determined by the sum of the products of reflection coefficients and molar concentrations of solutes. It follows that osmotic flow between two isosmotic solutions can only occur if they are separated by a permeable membrane and contain solute components with differing reflection coefficients. This is the basis of 'colloid' osmosis, similar to that induced by albumin across the capillary wall. The clinical application of this phenomenon to CAPD, of sustained ultrafiltration with physiological osmolality, is limited by an accumulation of maltose[22] but long-term studies are needed to evaluate this product fully.

Future solutions may well contain combinations of osmotic agents, e.g. amino acids or glucose (small molecules) and glucose polymer (large molecules) to yield initial high ultrafiltration from the small molecular weight agent which would be sustained by the large macro-molecules.

CAPD TECHNIQUE AND EQUIPMENT

The CAPD technique entails a 'closed system' whereby fluid is initially drained into the peritoneal cavity and drained out into the same bag after a dwell period (Figure 1.4). The spent bag is exchanged with a new one by a non-touch clean technique; this is done three to four times a day (up to 1500 exchanges per year). In order to prevent touch contamination various connection devices have been developed; hitherto none have eliminated peritonitis[25]. A major departure from the above technique was the development of the 'Y' system by Italian

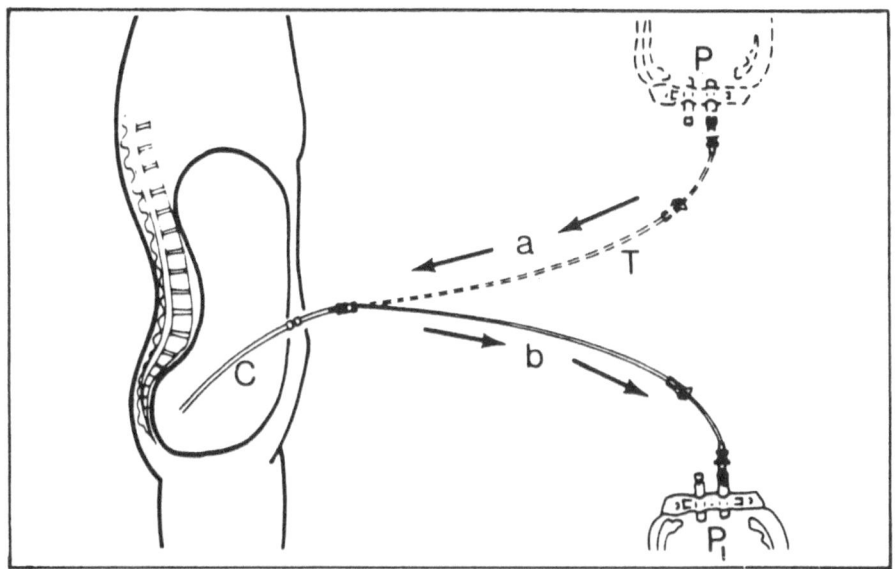

FIGURE 1.4 The CAPD system as widely practised by most CAPD patients. Only one bag (P) is used and kept attached to the Tenckhoff catheter (C) via a transfer set (T) at all times. Fluid is drained in via route (a) after the transfer set has been attached to a new bag P. After a dwell of 4 to 8 hours the dialysate is drained into the same bag by gravity. The 'Y' system utilizes a disposable double bag ($P P_1$) attached to the catheter (C) via a Y piece. At the time of an exchange this double bag system is connected to C, which is clamped off. Fresh fluid from P (15–30 ml) is flushed through the Y (if it contains disinfectant) into the empty bag P_1 (a–b). Dialysate from the peritoneal cavity is drained into P_1 before fresh fluid from P is drained into the patient. At the end of the procedure the bags and lines are disposed of and the catheter (or Y piece) capped

workers[26]. This entails drainage of the effluent after the connection is made with a new bag thereby enabling any touch contamination to be 'flushed' out before new fluid is drained into the peritoneal cavity. (Figure 1.4). The Y piece is filled with a disinfectant. This system has had a considerable effect in reducing peritonitis rates.

Peritoneal access is achieved by silicon catheters upon which the success of the CAPD technique depends. To date, no one type of catheter has proven superior to any other and this remains a weak point in the entire technique. The major problems with catheters are

TABLE 1.1   Catheter related problems

	Problem/solution
1. *Material*	
Silicon rubber, dacron cuffs	Allows ingrowth of bacteria and production of extracellular slime substance
2. *Insertion*	
Midline or lateral	Midline – prone to hernias and fluid leaks
Exit site and tunnel	Exit cuff erosion less when placed 2 cm from exit
	Exit pointing caudally to minimize exit infection (Swan neck catheter)
3. *Catheter complications*	
Fluid leak	*Early* – related to insertion and break-in technique, lateral insertion minimizes this
	Late – requires catheter replacement
Catheter obstruction	Constipation – relief of constipation Fibrin – use heparin/urokinase Displaced tip – reposition if possible Omental wrapping – replacement with omentectomy

Hernias
   Open processus vaginalis
     Right-sided hydrothorax
	Surgical approach to cure

4. *Unanswered questions on catheters*
   One or two cuffs
   Midline/lateral
   Open or closed insertion
   Type of catheter
   Constant catheter movement – 'pulling etc. at exchanges'? allows ingrowth of bacteria	

5. *Break-in technique* – 24 h post-op small cycle (500 ml) lavage
              – no PD for 7 days
              – beyond this increasing volume with CAPD cycles	

outlined in Table 1.1 which also lists the unanswered questions on catheter design, placement and postoperative use[27]. It would seem that lateral placement of a double cuff catheter through the rectus muscle with the catheter brought out such that the exit points caudally is most likely to minimize complications.

CLINICAL RESULTS

The relative advantages and disadvantages of CAPD as compared to haemodialysis and intermittent peritoneal dialysis are shown in Table 1.2.

TABLE 1.2   Relative advantages and disadvantages of CAPD as compared to haemodialysis and IPD

Advantages	Disadvantages
1. Well being	1. Peritonitis
2. Easier diet, fluid management, freedom to travel	2. Mechanical problems with catheters and connectors
3. Steady state biochemistry and improved 'middle molecule' removal	3. Hernias
	4. Patient dislikes 'burn out'
	5. ? Malnutrition
4. Improved anaemia and control of hypertension	6. Obesity and hyperlipidaemia
	7. Loss of ultrafiltration and peritoneal clearances
5. More appropriate for children, elderly, diabetics	8. Peritoneal sclerosis
6. Lower cost	
7. Improved bone disease	

Control of uraemia, fluid and electrolytes

CAPD unquestionably works and in the majority of patients produces good biochemical control. Since it is a continuous therapy, it provides steady state blood values for electrolytes and nitrogenous waste products. The precise blood levels will depend on the residual kidney function, the daily dialysate effluent volume and the production of

11

waste products, which in part reflect the dietary intake (see section on nutrition). Blood urea and creatinine concentrations of 20–30 mmol/l and 1000 μmol/l respectively are readily achieved. Disequilibrium is rare in CAPD. With judicious use of hypertonic peritoneal dialysis fluid, adequate amounts of sodium and water are removed; this has a bearing on blood pressure control. Likewise, potassium control is easy and hyperkalaemia is rare; this may be related to increased excretion of potassium via the faeces.[28] With a peritoneal dialysis fluid lactate concentration of 35 mmol/l, most patients are in a negative peritoneal bicarbonate balance and a slight metabolic acidosis is common[29]. This can be corrected by using a slightly more concentrated lactate solution of 40 mmol/l. Hypermagnesaemia is common using a concentration of 0.75 mmol/l in the PD fluid[29] but can be brought within the normal range by lowering the concentration of magnesium to 0.25 mmol/l[30].

Anaemia and hypertension

An increase in the well-being of patients after starting CAPD is probably, in part, due to the rise in haematocrit, which occurs within a few months of treatment. This is related to an increase in the red cell mass after six months[31]. The improvement, however, is not sustained long term and eventually comparable levels of haemoglobin to those on haemodialysis are observed[32]. Although the main reason for the anaemia of chronic renal failure remains the deficiency of erythropoietin, red cell survival is also important; the latter shows some improvement on CAPD and may be an important reason for the increase in red cell mass[32]. Iron utilization studies and an increase in the proliferation of bone marrow erythroid progenitor cells confirm the improvement in erythropoiesis after starting CAPD [33]. Whether this is related to an increased erythropoietin production or better removal of its inhibitors is uncertain; erythropoietin levels show no rise with time on CAPD. Studies on inhibitors of erythropoiesis *in vitro* (based on the effects of uraemic serum on erythroid progenitor cells) reveal an inverse relationship between haematocrit and inhibitors which are thought to be of 'middle molecule' size[34]. In addition, a direct relationship between haematocrit and peritoneal clearance of middle molecules has been demonstrated[35]. Overall, there appears to be an early and significant increase in the haematocrit, but long-term studies do not appear to show significantly better haemoglobin values than those achieved by haemodialysis patients.

During CAPD the ease with which sodium and water can be removed has led to the belief that hypertension is more readily controlled than on haemodialysis, where greater dietary sodium and water restriction is necessary. Studies have shown that blood pressure in patients on CAPD is elevated above normal and greater than in haemodialysis patients with similar elevations of plasma renin activity and aldosterone in both dialysis groups[36]. These two hormones, as well as the mean exchangeable sodium, therefore appeared not to have a direct or exclusive effect on blood pressure in CAPD patients. Symptomatic postural hypotension occurs in a small proportion of non-diabetic CAPD patients (especially the elderly) and is usually associated with sodium depletion and the use of low sodium dialysis fluid.

Renal osteodystrophy

Approximately 10% of patients reaching end-stage renal failure have evidence of hyperparathyroid bone disease. The introduction of CAPD influenced this status by altering the complex inter-relationship between calcium, phosphate, parathyroid hormone (PTH) and vitamin D. Using 1.36% glucose peritoneal dialysis solution (1.75 mmol calcium concentration) a positive calcium balance is achieved; net calcium transfer depends on plasma ionized calcium levels[28].

With a dietary intake of 800–1200 mg daily of phosphate, there would still be a need to remove 100–200 mg by the use of oral phosphate binding agents, assuming a 50% gut absorption and 250–350 mg removed in the dialysate[37]. CAPD does normalize serum total and ionized calcium levels: the overall effect of these changes on PTH is controversial as levels are either reported to be elevated or decreased with time[38]. What is becoming apparent is that suppression of PTH activity may only be brought about by high normal serum ionized calcium levels in conjunction with normal phosphate levels, suggesting a higher set point for calcium regulated PTH secretion[38,39]. To produce such high normal ionized calcium levels either oral calcium supplementation is necessary or the PD calcium concentration has to be increased. The former approach is more attractive; using oral calcium carbonate (up to 9 g daily) there is the added advantage of phosphate binding (if given at meal times) thus obviating the need for aluminium containing compounds. The dangers are hypercalcaemia and metastatic calcification, both of which have been reported[38,40]. Although earlier reports[40] suggested lower levels of 25-OHD$_3$ due to losses in the peritoneal fluid, this has not been substantiated in later studies; 1,25-OHD$_3$ levels are low. Vitamin D therapy is indicated for hypocalcaemia and hyperparathyroid bone disease.

There are few studies of a sufficiently large group of patients observed for suffcient length of time to draw any firm conclusions on the effect of these measures on renal osteodystrophy. The Newcastle group have shown consistent improvement for up to three years of CAPD on histological osteitis fibrosa[40] while Delmez et al. believe this is certainly possible in at least 75% of all patients treated on CAPD[41] where there is a concomitant decline in PTH levels. Non-aluminium related osteomalacia is readily cured by CAPD[42].

Aluminium toxicity in patients on CAPD is not a major problem and accumulation is almost invariably related to oral ingestion in the form of aluminium-containing phosphate binding agents, now that manufacturers can ensure that PD solution levels are less than $10\,\mu g/1$. Even without aluminium exposure, steady state serum aluminium levels of $30–40\,\mu g/1$ have been reported[42]. Whether these are toxic in the long term is still unknown; aluminium-related osteomalacia is uncommon, though reported, and can be treated effectively by either intravenous or intraperitoneal administration of desferrioxamine[43].

Overall, renal bone disease can be prevented by maintaining sufficiently high normal calcium concentrations to suppress PTH levels. This can be achieved by oral calcium carbonate which also acts as a phosphate binding agent thus reducing the exposure to aluminium. Routine prophylactic vitamin D therapy carries the risk of hypercalcaemia and hyperphosphataemia but intraperitoneal 1,25-OHD$_3$ administration may suppress PTH without raising serum calcium levels[44] and this possibility needs further study.

14

Nutrition

Chronic renal failure is associated with a variety of metabolic and endocrine disturbances that contribute to protein energy malnutrition and protein wasting[45]. Dialysis alters these and the initial experience with CAPD revealed several favourable effects: patients thrived, body weight and haematocrit increased, biochemical control was good and this collectively suggested an anabolic state. However, with long-term CAPD, several harmful metabolic factors have emerged including inferior removal of small molecular weight nitrogenous waste products as compared to haemodialysis[10], continuous loss of proteins, amino acids and other nutrients into the dialysate[46], a continuous supply of glucose and lactate from the dialysis fluid and finally inadequate nutritional intakes in many CAPD patients. These observations raise questions about the long-term metabolic and nutritional consequences of CAPD, which might limit its widespread use[47].

Carbohydrate metabolism

Due to the hyperglycaemic stress of the continuous peritoneal absorption of 100–200 g glucose/day there is a tendency towards constantly elevated serum insulin levels. Overt diabetes is rare (but described) as CAPD does not lead to exhaustion of pancreatic cells. Single cycle studies using glucose as the osmotic agents have shown that CAPD not only results in the glucose/insulin disturbances already discussed but also leads to reduced gluconeogenesis, inhibition of lipolysis and suppression of ketogenesis; in addition, the elevated glucagon, alanine and lactate levels remain unchanged[48]. These changes may contribute to several potentially adverse metabolic and nutritional effects – reduced appetite, excessive weight gain, aggravation of serum lipid and lipoprotein abnormalities and alteration in amino acid metabolism[49].

Lipid metabolism

Uraemic hypertryglyceridaemia and dyslipoproteinaemia persist during CAPD. Lipid abnormalities are usually worsened during the initial months of treatment and the changes correlate with the peritoneal glucose load[49]. The hyperlipidaemic changes are due to concurrently increased lipid concentrations in the VLDL and LDL fractions, whereas changes in HDL are less well marked. Furthermore, these changes are more apparent in patients already hyperlipidaemic at the start of CAPD[50]. Long-term studies of patients on CAPD for more than five years show a similar pattern with only a moderate hypertriglyceridaemia (Lamiere, Belgium, unpublished observations). Most workers report that the ratios between LDL and HDL cholesterol and between VLDL + LDL and HDL increase significantly[49].

Obesity in CAPD

There are several reports of markedly increased body weight in some patients on CAPD; this, in part, is related to increased body fat as shown by increases in skinfold thickness[51] or increase in mean fat cell size[49]. Few patients, however, become overtly obese and most seem to return to their premorbid non-uraemic weight. This latter effect may be related to a decreased appetite from abdominal distension and delayed gastric emptying[52].

Protein and amino acid metabolism

The substantial loss of protein into the dialysate (5–15 g daily – doubled during episodes of peritonitis) is a major drawback. There are large inter-individual differences but in an individual losses are fairly constant. The major fractions found in the effluent are albumin (48–65%) and IgG (15%) but most proteins are lost and this depends on the molecular weight and size, peritoneal permeability and serum concentrations[53]. Despite this, most patients maintain stable total protein and albumin levels, although in the low normal range. Serum transferrin and C3 levels may even increase to normal during the initial anabolic months of CAPD. In addition, Kaysin and Schoenfeld[54] have reported plasma albumin mass, total albumin mass and distribution of albumin to be normal in CAPD.

Patients on CAPD exhibit plasma amino acid abnormalities that are similar to those in other uraemic patients; a decrease in total essential amino acids and the decreased ratios between valine/glycine and tyrosine/phenylalanine in part reflect losses in the dialysate of 1.2–3.4 g/day (29% essential; 57% of total nitrogenous losses)[49]. Muscle free amino acids are abnormal with reduced levels of tyrosine and taurine and increased levels of lysine, asparagine, aspartic acid, glutamic acid and citrulline[55].

During the first 6–12 months of CAPD there appears to be nitrogen equilibrium or protein nitrogen balance which correlates with weight gain, dietary protein and total energy intake. Although few patients develop overt protein malnutrition, except in severe peritonitis, there is a gradual reduction in nutritional intake with time with decreases in nitrogen balance after three years of CAPD [49]. Protein and calorie intake decline significantly (protein from 1.2 to less than 1 g/kg/day; calories from 35 to less than 30 kcal/kg/day).

Adequacy of dialysis and nutritional therapy

Adequacy of dialysis is still difficult to define and no one measure has proved acceptable. Urea, creatinine, albumin and haemoglobin concentrations are all influenced by nutritonal factors, protein in particular. Whereas there are some signs that CAPD provides adequate dialysis (improved platelet function, immunological competence and anaemia), other uraemic symptoms are not adequately controlled – increasing tiredness, insomnia, muscle weakness and anorexia, which in turn lead to inadequate nutrient intake. Single measurements of urea and creatinine are far from ideal in determining adequacy of dialysis or protein intake. To overcome this, use is made of the linear and predictable relationship between urea nitrogen appearance and total nitrogen output; thus dietary protein can be estimated assuming neutral nitrogen balance[56] (urea nitrogen appearance g/24 hours = urea nitrogen in dialysate and urine; $1 \text{ g N}_2 = 6.25 \text{ g}$ protein).

TABLE 1.3   Dietary nutritional requirements in CAPD

Energy	30–50 kcal/kg/day (including that from glucose absorption); 30–35 kcal/kg/day for obese patients
Protein	1.2 g/kg/day
Lipids	P:S ratio 1.5:1
Potassium[a]	60–80 mmol/day
Magnesium[a]	200–300 mg/day
Calcium[a]	1–4 g/day (including oral calcium supplements)
Phosphate	0.7–1.2 g/day
Vitamin/	Oral supplements: C (100–200 mg/day) B1 (10–40 mg/day) B6 (5–15 mg/day) Folic acid (0.5–1.0 mg/day)

[a] Using PD fluid with zero K, 0.75 mmol Mg, 1.75 mmol/L Ca

What then are the recommended dietary and nutritional requirements in CAPD patients? These are shown in Table 1.3. Individualized dietary prescriptions are necessary and *ad libitum* diets should definitely be discouraged. Anorexia and abdominal distension can be minimized by eating meals drained of fluid.

Peritonitis

Since the introduction of CAPD, peritonitis has remained the most significant complication accounting for considerable morbidity and causing many patients to be changed from CAPD to haemodialysis. Peritonitis rates have improved since the early days when bottled peritoneal dialysis fluid was used. This improvement is due not only to the superior equipment but also to a better understanding of the pathogenesis. Recent reports[26] raise the possibility that effective prevention of peritoneal infection may well become a reality in the not too distant future; an episode of peritonitis every 3–4 years in a patient's CAPD life is probably acceptable.

The clinical aspects of peritonitis complicating the course of CAPD have been thoroughly analysed[57] and differ from surgical or IPD peritonitis in several respects. These differences are related to the constant presence of fluid in the peritoneal cavity which is repeatedly drained. This situation not only leads to rapid dissemination of bacteria throughout the peritoneal cavity following apparently minor contamination but allows early detection of inflammation by the turbidity of the fluid. Bacteraemia following CAPD peritonitis is extremely rare and the confinement of infection to the peritoneal cavity allows direct therapy via anti-infectious agents added to fresh PD fluid. Finally CAPD peritonitis has a more benign prognosis than surgical peritonitis.

The definition and diagnosis of peritonitis are now fairly well agreed upon, although there is no universally accepted approach to its management. The predominance of skin commensals as infecting organisms has been amply confirmed and improvements in culture techniques have decreased the incidence of culture-negative peritonitis.

TABLE 1.4   Possible pathways for infection of peritoneal cavity

1. *Exogenous contamination through lumen of catheter*
    Bag exchange
    Transfer set exchange
    Injection of drugs
    Airborne contamination
    Defective PD system
    Accidental disconnections
    Infected PD fluid

2. *Exogenous contamination across abdominal wall*
    Exit site infection
    Dacron cuff and tunnel infection

3. *Endogenous contamination*
    Transcolonic migration of bacteria
    Intra-abdominal infected viscera
    Haematogenous
    Female genital tract

4. *Other routes*
    Lymphatics

Treatment strategies utilize intraperitoneal antibiotics with very little established role for oral therapy. Whilst there have been some advances in treatment policies, the more novel and exciting developments have been related to a greater understanding of the pathogenesis of peritonitis.

The factors which are important in causing CAPD peritonitis relate not only to the equipment, connectors and lines but to other less well defined entities such as patient training, medical and nursing competence, experience and enthusiasm, and a proper infrastructure to train patients. Contamination of the connector system during the exchange procedure remains the most important cause of peritonitis although the possible pathways of infection are many (Table 1.4). Developments so far have failed to eradicate the problem in spite of some clever innovations such as the ultraviolet sterilizing system, and the sterile connecting device. Italian workers using the Y system[26], which is now generally recognized as being superior to the standard set, have reported peritonitis rates of less than one episode/24 patient months.

Pathogenesis – catheter colonization

Peritonitis has a complex pathogenesis as confirmed by recent work. There is now considerable evidence to show that coagulase-negative staphylococci (in particular *Staphylococcus epidermidis*) are the major causative organisms in infections of prosthetic devices and intravascular catheters[58]. These organisms are able to adhere to and grow on polymer surfaces. In the course of surface colonization they produce an extracellular 'slime substance' resulting in the formation of a thick matrix with embedded staphylococcal layers. This slime substance or biofilm inhibits the chemotactic responses of neutrophils, proliferative responses of lymphocytes and opsonization of bacteria and may also serve as a penetration barrier to several antibiotics. Tenckhoff CAPD catheters have also been studied and scanning electron microscopy of the external and internal surfaces of such catheters which had been removed for various reasons revealed this biofilm with encased adherent bacterial microcolonies[59]. In addition, quantitative microbiological recovery methods in rabbits showed colonization of the external surface of the catheter in the subcutaneous tunnel by Gram-positive

20

cocci forming a continuous and coherent biofilm on the catheter surface. The film reached the external dacron cuff in an average of three days and penetrated it to reach the peritoneal portions of the catheter in an average of three weeks. This protective biofilm then comprised an inherently antibiotic-resistant reservoir of bacteria which could generate repeated episodes of peritonitis.

Why is it that all patients do not get peritonitis? One third of CAPD patients remain peritonitis free and a small proportion account for more than half the episodes. There are reports of bacteria being cultured from clear effluents[60] and evidence of bacteria multiplying within peritoneal macrophages[61]. In addition, half the episodes of peritonitis are related to non-*S. epidermidis* infections, arguing against all infections being related to the catheter. The answer to this question almost certainly lies in the failure of local host defence mechanisms which must be overwhelmed by bacteria (a large enough innoculum at bag exchanges or from catheter surfaces) to produce peritonitis.

Host defence mechanism

Normal peritoneal defence resides in the lymphatics and cellular mechanisms. The overall cellular content of PD effluents is roughly 8.5 million cells per exchange[62], 90% of which are viable and roughly half display the characteristics of peritoneal macrophages. Although these cells exhibit bacterial phagocytic activity equal to blood neutrophils, their low concentration increases the chance of infection. The phagocytic process, in addition, involves chemotaxis and opsonization. Opsonins are substances which act as ligands to facilitate bacterial attachment to phagocytic cells. The two most important are IgG (heat stable – important for Gram-positive organisms) and C3 (heat stable – and involved with Gram-negative bacteria). The complete phagocytic process involves interleukin 1 and interleukin 2 with the final common path involving γ-interferon (Figure 1.5). Keane *et al.*[63] have shown deficiency of the opsonic activity and demonstrated a significant correlation with the incidence of peritonitis. These results have been confirmed by others. In addition, Lamperi and Carozzi[64] have recently shown that γ-interferon can enhance peritoneal macrophage antibacterial activities. In a group of patients with a high peritonitis rate

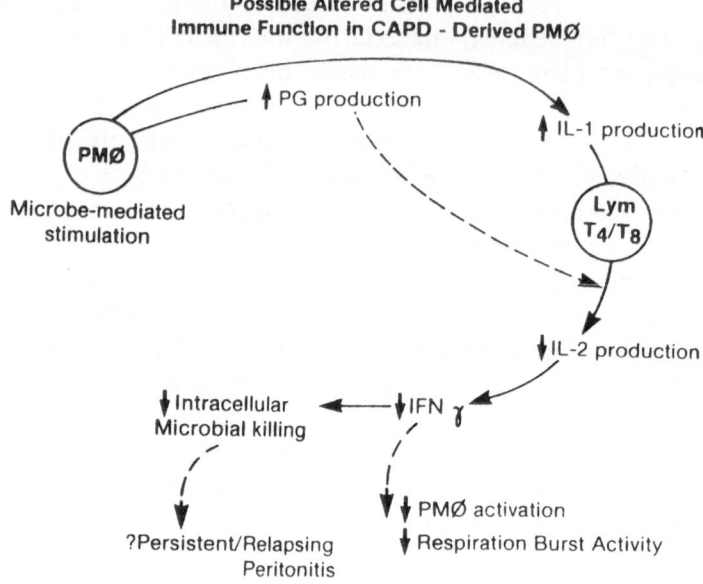

Possible Altered Cell Mediated Immune Function in CAPD - Derived PMØ

FIGURE 1.5 Possible altered cell-mediated immune function in CAPD derived peritoneal macrophages (PM). PG = prostaglandin; IFN = γ-interferon; Lym = lymphocytes; → = stimulation; -- → = some degree of inhibition

they showed a lack of IgG-Fc receptors with a decrease in macrophage oxidative metabolism and killing, features that were reversed by incubation *in vitro* with γ-interferon. These results paved the way for stimulating heat-stable opsonic activity by adding IgG to PD fluid; when given every three weeks to patients with a high peritonitis rate, the significant reduction in peritonitis achieved[65] was related to increased γ-interferon levels in the PD effluent. Additional research is required in this field, for example to determine which subclasses of IgG are important.

The risk of developing peritonitis, therefore, rests on a delicate balance between colonization of the CAPD system, the quantity of bacteria invading the peritoneal cavity and the local peritoneal host defence mechanism. Improvement in catheter design, stimulating the local host defences and developing staphylococcal vaccines[66] may well reduce the incidence of peritonitis to acceptable levels. It is interesting to speculate why the 'Y' system developed by the Italians and incorporating disinfectant gives superior results. Other than the 'flush' theory, it may be that the hypochlorite disinfectant, which is a per-oxide-like material, may be releasing hydrogen peroxide which can remove the biofilm on catheters and prevent its formation; this assumes that minute quantities do go past the clamp into the catheters at exchanges.

The development of the vaccine has been facilitated by the studies of Ballardie et al.[66] who have shown a rise of antibodies to coagulase-negative staphylococci following episodes of peritonitis. The half-life of these antibodies is considerable and may prevent subsequent episodes of infection. Vaccines against S. aureus infection have been tried but experience to date is preliminary, limited and anecdotal.

Consequences of peritonitis

During episodes of peritonitis, there are decreases in ultrafiltration, increases in the peritoneal clearances of urea and enhanced protein losses. Peritoneal inflammation is associated with a rich exudate and depressed fibrinolytic activity which result in a short-lived loss of ultrafiltration; this reverts to normal when the infection is cured. Repeated episodes of peritonitis may lead to adhesions, sclerosis and loss of ultrafiltration – any of which may be a reason for discontinuing CAPD. Peritonitis remains the major cause of drop-out from CAPD.

Loss of ultrafiltration and peritoneal sclerosis

A major concern of nephrologists relates to the long-term viability of the peritoneum which nature did not evolve for the purpose of dialysis! CAPD constantly exposes the delicate peritoneal membrane to unphysiological solutions, containing substances known to be poten-tially harmful. Although some studies have shown preservation of mass transfer coefficients and peritoneal clearances after several years of CAPD[67], the loss of ultrafiltration capacity[68] and development of sclerosing encapsulating peritonitis[69] are worrying complications. Whilst these complications are at present infrequent, workers are concerned about the viability of the peritoneal membrane during CAPD continuing for 10 years or more.

Sheldon[70] has recently put forward a hypothesis to explain the development of these two problems. He suggests that the peritoneal macrophages are in a state of 'over-stimulation' from exogenous factors such as peritoneal dialysis fluid, glucose metabolites, peritonitis, acetate and disinfectants. These macrophages release interleukin 1, which at the peritoneal level stimulates fibroblasts to produce more collagen and initiate fibrosis; it also induces endothelial cells to release prostacyclin which, being a vasodilator, leads to a rapid loss of glucose gradient and then to a loss of ultrafiltration with time[71]. Recent studies of lymphatic reabsorption suggest that this factor may be of considerable significance[18] especially in patients with 'virgin' abdomens who have poor ultrafiltration from the start of CAPD.

There are permeability changes in patients who suffer loss of ultrafiltration and Verger[72] has delineated two patterns. Type I corresponds to a hyperpermeable membrane (as assessed by D/P ratio of glucose and urea) which, histologically, shows loss of mesothelial microvilli and increased cell separation. Type II occurs when the permeability is low and is associated with multiple adhesions or sclerosing encapsulating peritonitis. Of particular importance is the observation that Type I is reversible on cessation of peritoneal dialysis but, if continued, Type II changes, which are irreversible, may well supervene[73]. Dobbie et al. have put forward a theory, based on examination of histological sections[4,74], to account for loss of ultrafiltration and fibrosis. They point to the irreversibility of damage observed after repeated episodes of peritonitis from the outpouring of fibrinous exudate, secondary to changes mediated by mast cells which gather in large numbers at the site of injury and release their polypeptides and nucleotides. Finally, the constant use of hypertonic solutions may have a deleterious effect on the mesothelium and lead to loss of ultrafiltration[75].

Whatever the mechanism the end result of the thickening of the peritoneum is sclerosing encapsulating peritonitis; 85 cases of this lethal condition have been described[60]. This disease is characterized by the development of a 'new membrane' that encases, wholly or partially, the small bowel such that the appearance resembles a cocoon. Repeated attacks of peritonitis, use of acetate in PD fluid and disinfectants (especially chlorhexidine) are believed to be important causative factors.

Is there any cure for loss of ultrafiltration? Other than discontinuing CAPD, using less hypertonic solutions and leaving the peritoneum empty overnight to allow the mesothelium to regenerate, there is no solution. However, initial preliminary work by Lamperi and Carozzi[76] on the use of calcium channel antagonists to improve ultrafiltration is fascinating. In some CAPD patients, peritoneal macrophages and lymphocytes become hyperactivated by a calcium-dependent mechanism and secrete large amounts of lympho-monokines (interleukin 1 and γ-interferon), which stimulate peritoneal fibroblast proliferation. Calcium channel antagonist block endocellular calcium leading to a reversal of these abnormalities.

THE USE AND OUTCOME OF CAPD

The number of patients on CAPD over the last decade has shown a dramatic but steady increase throughout the world. The number of CAPD patients as a percentage of the total dialysis population varies from country to country (Figure 1.6). Despite this phenomenal growth in its use the long-term progress of patients on CAPD is still uncertain[77]. The earlier reports from the European Dialysis and Transplant Registry on patient survival and technique 'drop-out' rates were such that only a quarter of the patients remained on CAPD after two years[78]. These results undoubtedly reflected a learning phase and did not differ markedly from the initial experience of haemodialysis 20 years earlier.

Recent reports are, however, more encouraging with medium-term survival up to five years being comparable to that on haemodialysis. Most units have a few patients who are now into their seventh or eighth year of treatment by CAPD but the numbers are small.

The largest database on CAPD in the world is that of the National Institutes of Health in the USA. This CAPD registry has follow-up data on over 16000 patients[79]. The most recent analysis reveals a cumulative probability of death after three years of 42%, that of transfer to haemodialysis or IPD of 44% and a 'drop-out' (for any reason including death and transplantation) probability of 75% after

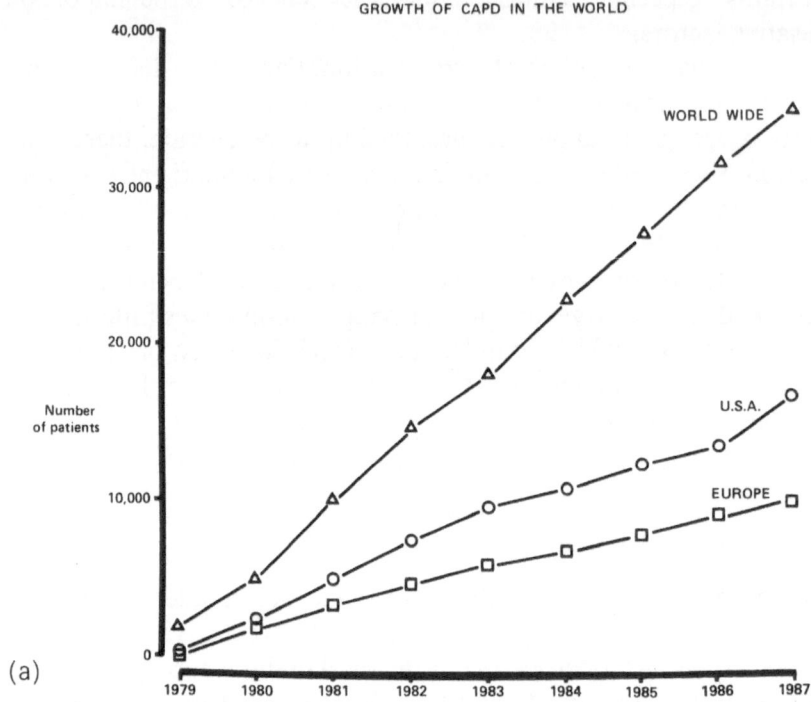

(a)

FIGURE 1.6   (a) The number of patients on therapy with CAPD, in the world, USA and Europe. (b) Percentage of dialysis patients on CAPD in various countries; 11% of dialysis population was managed by CAPD as at end of 1986. (Data provided by Travenol)

three years. Peritonitis (found in 29% of patients) was the commonest cause of transfer to haemodialysis or IPD. The cumulative probability of death increased two-fold if the patients were older than 60 years or were diabetics; the latter group formed 31% of all patients accepted for CAPD in 1986.

No such recent data on the outcome of CAPD are available from the EDTA Registry. The Canadian Renal Failure Registry, established in 1981, has reported on its five year experience[80] that there is an age-related difference in survival and a statistically significant difference in overall survival between diabetic and non-diabetic patients.

In the UK, two studies have been conducted. One was a prospective study on the outcome of patients on CAPD and HD[81]. The four year

26

% CAPD PATIENTS

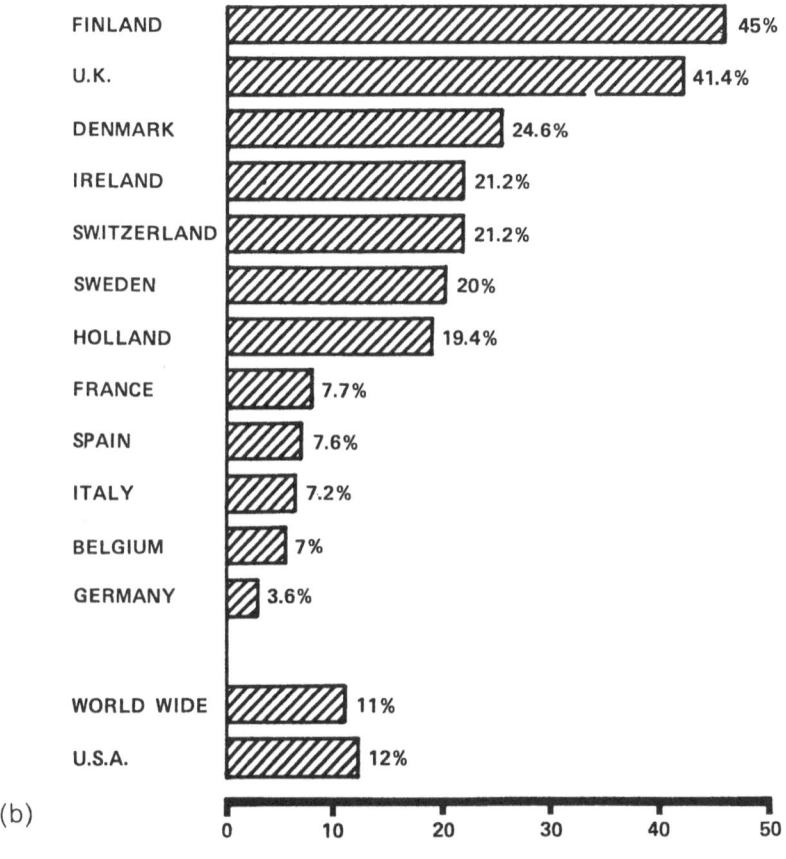

(b)

analysis has revealed that CAPD is now used twice as often as HD as the first line dialysis therapy; moreover, those patients with risk factors (age > 60, diabetics, cardio/cerebrovascular disease) tended to be accepted preferentially for CAPD. In spite of this bias in selection policy patient survival was equivalent in the two groups (72% HD, 64% CAPD at 4 years) although Cox multivariate analysis showed that the presence of risk factors adversely affected survival. The major cause of 'drop-out' was a desirable one – successful transplantation – whilst

27

the technique survival (death and transplantation excluded as lost to follow-up) was inferior in the CAPD group (91% HD, 61% CAPD). Peritonitis was the reason for transfer to HD in just under half those who changed. Interestingly, morbidity as reflected by hospitalization was similar (HD 12.8 days/patient year; CAPD 14.7 days/patient year); this amounted to a requirement of 6–8 back-up beds in a large CAPD programme of 100 patients. The HD back-up for temporary or permanent change amounted to 1–2 HD stations.

The other UK study was a retrospective one involving four centres which detailed the outcome of CAPD on patients who started treatment before 1981. After four years, only 19% were still on CAPD[82]. Studies from individual centres support these multicentre analyses. Indeed, the report on the selection-adjusted comparison of life expectancy for patients on CAPD, HD and transplantation showed that the risks in these categories did not differ significantly and thus suggested that CAPD was at least as effective at preserving life[83].

Technique failure rate may well be higher than in HD but undoubtedly reflects a wide variation in the deployment of CAPD in individual centres. Reported series with defined 'standardized' populations (15–55 years, primary renal disease, no cardiovascular or other serious complications) showed differences in terms of patient selection, social and medical factors at the start of treatment[84]. The value of such comparisons between CAPD and HD is therefore limited and statistical assessment dubious.

PATIENT SELECTION AND QUALITY OF LIFE

Patients can be maintained in excellent condition at least in the short term. Certain patients fare better on this treatment than on HD and factors that need to be taken into account on selecting patients for CAPD are shown in Table 1.5. Patients with diabetes mellitus or cardiovascular disease, small children and the elderly do well on CAPD. Renal transplantation has an important bearing on the choice of type of dialysis for a patient in ESRF. For those suitable, CAPD before transplantation would seem to be the most appropriate approach. Home haemodialysis could then be reserved for those for whom transplantation is impossible or is likely to be delayed beyond

TABLE 1.5   Factors influencing choice of CAPD in new patients

Medical factors	Psychosocial factors
Age	Patient preference
Ischaemic heart disease	Motivation
Diabetes mellitus	Compliance
Ease of transplantation	Family support
Extensive abdominal surgery	Distance from centre
Blindness	Occupation
Severe pulmonary disease	Concern with body image
Peripheral vascular disease	Travel
Lumbar disc problems	
Extensive diverticulitis?	

two or three years. Many highly sensitized patients may fall into this category. Those patients unable to undertake home dialysis would require in-centre hospital dialysis for which facilities in the UK are limited. This approach presupposes that availability of kidneys and transplantation results are both good and that grafts are allocated on the basis of HLA matching[84].

What about the quality of life achieved on CAPD? Several studies have addressed this question. A multicentre report in the USA[85] involving 859 patients on renal replacement therapy (80 CAPD) showed that 79% of transplant recipients were able to function at nearly 'normal' levels as opposed to 47.5% for CAPD   and 59% for home haemodialysis patients. In-centre haemodialysis patients appeared to fare least well. On three subjective measures (life satisfaction, well-being and psychological effect), the transplant patients had a higher quality of life than those receiving treatment in hospital and perceived their life-style to be only slightly inferior to that of the general population.

A study of patients from Manchester Royal Infirmary and Oxford Renal Units reached similar conclusions[86]; patients were classified into those above and below 60 years with or without risk factors. The patients that did least well were males below 60 years with risk factors. Employment suffered once patients started treatment. Fragola et al.[87] found that only 27% of patients were able to continue the job they held before starting CAPD, while the Oxford–Manchester study showed that only half of those previously employed or fit to work were able to do so after beginning treatment. In the USA study[84], only 25% of those initially employed continued to work after starting CAPD compared with 60% of patients on home haemodialysis and 75% of transplant recipients. These differences almost certainly reflect patient selection with a bias towards placing high-risk patients on CAPD or hospital haemodialysis. Although these patients are able to adapt to very adverse life circumstances, objective evidence of successful rehabilitation is rare except for transplant recipients and some home haemodialysis patients.

With the introduction of CAPD into the UK many patients have been accepted for treatment who would have previouly been denied therapy. The doubling of the acceptance rate for new patients achieved in the last five years has been primarily related to CAPD. There is no doubt about the efficacy of CAPD in the short term (up to five years) but long-term results are awaited. Improvements in equipment, development of alternative osmotic agents to glucose, and a better understanding of the role of host defence will minimize complications, diminish the potentially deleterious effect of continuous CAPD on the peritoneum and improve both patient survival and quality of life. CAPD is here to stay and one can be cautiously optimistic about its future.

REFERENCES

1. Popovich, R. P., Moncrief, J. W., Decherd, J. F., Bomar, J. B., Pyle, W. K. (1976). The definition of a novel portable/wearable equilibrium dialysis technique. *Trans. Am. Soc. Artif. Int. Organs,* **5,** 64
2. Gokal, R. (1986). Historical development and clinical use of continuous ambulatory peritoneal dialysis. In Gokal, R. (ed) *Continuous Ambulatory Peritoneal Dialysis*, pp. 1–13. (Edinburgh: Churchill Livingstone)
3. Di Paolo, N., Buoncristiani, U., Capotondo, L., Gaggiotti, E., De Mia, M., Rossi, P., Sansoni, E., Bernini, M. (1986). Phosphatidylcholine and peritoneal transport during PD. *Nephron,* **44,** 365–370
4. Dobbie, J. W., Zaki, M., Wilson, L. (1981). Ultrastructural studies on the peritoneum with special reference to CAPD. *Scot. Med. J.,* **26,** 213–223
5. Verger, C., Luger, A., Moore, J. U., Nolph, K. D. (1983). Acute changes in peritoneal morphology and transport properties with infectious peritonitis and mechanical injury. *Kidney Int.,* **23,** 823–831
6. Nolph, K. D., Miller, F., Rubin, J., Popovich, R. (1980). New directions in peritoneal dialysis concepts and applications. *Kidney Int.,* **18,** S111–6 (Suppl 10)
7. Henderson, L. W. (1966). Peritoneal ultrafiltration dialysis: enhanced urea transfer using hypertonic peritoneal fluid. *J. Clin. Invest.,* **45,** 950–955

8. Kallen, R. J. (1966). A method for approximating the efficacy of peritoneal dialysis for uraemia. *Am. J. Dis. Child.*, **3**, 156–160
9. Dedrick, R. L., Flessner, M. F., Collins, J. M., Schultz, J. S. (1982). Is the peritoneum a membrane? *ASAIO J.*, **5**, 1–8
10. Popovich, R. P., Pyle, W. K., Hiatt, M. P., McCollough, W. S. Moncrief, J. W. (1980). Metabolite transport kinetics in peritoneal dialysis. In Legrain, M. (ed) *Continuous Ambulatory Peritoneal Dialysis*, pp. 28–33. (Amsterdam: Excerpta Medica)
11. Spencer, P. C., Farrell, P. C. (1986). Solute and water transfer kinetics in CAPD. In Gokal, R. (ed) *Continuous Ambulatory Peritoneal Dialysis*, pp. 38–55. (Edinburgh: Churchill Livingstone)
12. DePaepe, M., Kips, J., Belpairi, F., Lamiere, N. (1986). Comparison of different volume markers in peritoneal dialysis. In Maher, J.F. Winchester, J.F. (eds) *Frontiers in Peritoneal Dialysis*, pp. 279–283. (New York: Field Richard Assoc.)
13. Nolph, K. D. (1983). Solute and urate transport during peritoneal dialysis. *Perspect Peritoneal Dialysis*, **1**, 4–8
14. Shear, L., Swartz, C., Shinaberger, J. H., Barry, K. G. (1965). Kinetics of peritoneal fluid absorption in adult man. *N. Engl. J. Med.*, **272**, 123–6
15. Daugirdas, J. T., Ing, T. S., Gandhi, V. C., Hano, J. S., Chen, W. T., Yuan, L. (1980). Kinetics of peritoneal fluid absorption in patients with chronic renal failure. *J. Lab. Clin. Med.*, **95**, 351–361
16. Rippe, B., Stelin, G., Ahlen, J. (1986). Lymph flow from the peritoneal cavity in CAPD patients. In Maher, J. F., Winchester, J. F. (eds) *Frontiers in Peritoneal Dialysis*, pp. 24–30. (New York: Field Rich and Assoc.)
17. Courtice, F. C., Steinbech, A. W. (1951). The effects of lymphatic obstruction and of posture on the absorption of protein from peritoneal cavity. *Aust. J. Exp. Biol. Med. Sci.*, **29**, 451–458
18. Mactier, R. A., Khanna, R., Twardowski, Z., Nolph, K. D. (1987). Contribution of lymphatic absorption to loss of ultrafiltration and solute clearances in CAPD. *J. Clin. Invest.*, **80**, 1311–1316
19. Twardowski, Z., Khanna, R., Nolph, K. D. (1986). Osmotic agents and ultrafiltration in peritoneal dialysis. *Nephron*, **42**, 93–101
20. Han, H., Kessel, M. (1987). Aspects of new solutions for peritoneal dialysis. *Nephrol. Dial. Transplant.*, **2**, 67–72
21. Mistry, C. D., Mallick, N. P., Gokal, R. (1986). The use of large molecular weight glucose polymer (MW 20 000) as an osmotic agent in CAPD. In Khanna, R. *et al.* (eds) *Advances in Continuous Ambulatory Peritoneal Dialysis 1986*, pp. 7–11. (Toronto: Univ. of Toronto Press)
22. Mistry, C. D., Mallick, N. P., Gokal, R. (1985). The advantages of glucose polymer as an osmotic agent in CAPD. *Proc. Eur. Dial. Transplant Assoc.*, **22**, 415–420
23. Khanna, R., Mactier, R., Twardowski, Z., Nolph, K. D. (1986). Peritoneal cavity lymphatics. *Perit. Dial. Bull.*, **6**, 113–121
24. Caseley-Smith, J. R. (1964). Endothelial permeability. The passage of particles into and out of diaphragmatic lymphatics. *Q.J. Exp. Physiol.*, **49**, 365–383
25. Winchester, J. F. (1986). CAPD systems and solutions. In Gokal, R. (ed) *Continuous Ambulatory Peritoneal Dialysis*, pp. 94–109. (Edinburgh: Churchill Livingstone)
26. Maiorca, R., Cantaluppi, A., Cancarini, G. C., Scalamogna, A., Broccoli, R.,

26. Maiorca, R., Cantaluppi, A., Cancarini, G. C., Scalamogna, A., Broccoli, R., Rasiani, Bras, S., Ponticelli, C. (1983). Prospective controlled trial of a Y connector and disinfectant to prevent peritonitis in CAPD. *Lancet*, **2**, 642–4
27. Veitch, P. (1986). Surgical aspects of CAPD. In Gokal, R. (ed) *Continuous Ambulatory Peritoneal Dialysis*, pp. 110–144. (Edinburgh: Churchill Livingstone)
28. Blumenkrantz, M., Kopple, J., Moran, J. (1982). Metabolic balance studies and dietary protein requirements in CAPD. *Kidney Int.*, **21**, 849–58
29. Gokal, R. (1982). Renal osteodystrophy in CAPD. *Perit. Dial. Bull.*, **2**, 111–115
30. Nolph, K. D., Prowant, B., Serkes, K. D., Morgan, L., Baker, B., Charytan, C., Gham, K., Hamburger, R., Husserl, F., Kleit, S., McGuiness, J., Moore, H., Warren, T. (1983). Multicentre evaluation of a new peritoneal dialysis solution with a high lactate and a low magnesium concentration. *Perit. Dial. Bull.*, **3**, 63–65
31. DePaepe, M. B. J., Schelstraete, K. H. G., Ringoir, S. M., Lamiere, N. H. (1983). Influence of CAPD on the anaemia of end stage renal disease. *Kidney Int.*, **23**, 744–748
32. Salahudeen, A. K., Keavy, P. M., Hawkins, T., Wilkinson, R. (1983). Is anaemia during CAPD really better than during haemodialysis? *Lancet*, **2**, 1046–1049
33. Lamperi, S., Carozzi, S. (1983). *In vitro* and *in vivo* studies of erythropoiesis during CAPD. *Perit. Dial. Bull.*, **3**, 94–96
34. McGonigle, R. J. S., Husserl, F., Wallen, J. D., Fisher, J. W. (1984). Haemodialysis and CAPD effects on erythopoiesis in renal failure. *Kidney Int.*, **25**, 430–436
35. Lamperi, S., Carozzi, S., Icardi, A. (1983). Improvement of erythropoiesis in uraemic patients on CAPD. *Int. J. Artif. Organs*, **6**, 191–194
36. Youmbissi, J., Sellars, L., Shore, A. C., Poon, T., Wilkinson, R. (1986). Blood pressure on CAPD: relationship to sodium status, renin and aldosterone compared with haemodialysis. In Maher, J. F., Winchester, J. F. (ed) *Frontiers in Peritoneal Dialysis*, pp. 450–455. (New York: Field Rich and Assoc)
37. Delmez, J. A., Slatopolsky, E., Martin, K. J., Gearing, B. N., Harler, H. R. (1982). Minerals, vitamin D and parathyroid hormone in CAPD. *Kidney Int.*, **21**, 862–867
38. Gokal, R. (1986). Renal osteodystrophy and aluminium status in CAPD patients. In La Greca, G., Fabris, A., Ronco, C. (eds) *Peritoneal Dialysis II*, pp. 225–228. (Milan: Wichtig Editore)
39. Slatopolsky, E., Martin, K. J., Mirrissey, J. J., Hruska, K. A. (1985). Parathyroid hormone: alteration in CRF. In Robinson, R. R. (ed) *Nephrology Vol. II*, pp. 1292–1304. (New York. Springer-Verlag)
40. Cassidy, M. J. D., Owen, J. P., Ellis, H. A., Dewar, J., Robinson, C. J., Wilkinson, R., Ward, M. K., Kerr, D. N. S. (1985). Renal osteodystrophy and metastatic calcification in long term CAPD. *Q. J. Med.*, **213**, 29–48
41. Delmez, J. A., Fallon, M. D., Bergfeld, M. A., Gearing, B. K., Dougan, C. S., Teitelbaum, S. L. (1986). CAPD and bone. *Kidney Int.*, **30**, 379–384
42. Gokal, R., Ramos, J. M., Ellis, H. A. (1983). Histological renal osteodystrophy and 25-hydroxycholecalciferol and aluminium levels in patients in CAPD. *Kidney Int.*, **23**, 15–21
43. Hercz, G., Salusky, L. B., Norris, K. C., Fine, R. N., Coburn, J. W. (1986). Aluminium removal by peritoneal dialysis: intravenous vs intraperitoneal desferoxamine. *Kidney Int.*, **30**, 944–948
44. Delmez, J. A., Gearing, B. N. (1987). Renal osteodystrophy and aluminium bone disease in CAPD patients. In Khanna, K. (ed) *Advances in CAPD, 1987*, pp. 38–45 (Toronto: University of Toronto Press)

45. Emmanuel, D. S., Lindheimer, M. D., Katz, A. (1981). Metabolic and endocrine abnormalities in chronic renal failure. In Brenner, B. M., Stein, J. H. (eds) *Chronic Renal Failure*, pp. 46-83. (New York: Churchill Livingstone)
46. Blumenkrantz, M. J., Gahl, G. M., Kopple, J. D., Kamdar, A., Jones, M., Kessel, M., Coburn, J. W. (1981). Protein losses during peritoneal dialysis. *Kidney Int.*, **19**, 593-602
47. Lindholm, B., Alverstrand, A., Norbeck, H. E., Tranoeus, A., Bergstrom, J. (1984). Long-term metabolic consequence of CAPD. In Robinson, R.R. (ed) *Nephrology*, Vol. II, pp. 1611-1626. (New York: Springer-Verlag)
48. Heaton, A., Johnston, D. G., Burren, J. M., Orskow, H., Ward, M. K., Alberti, K. G. M. Kerr, D. N. S. (1983). Carbohydrate and lipid metabolism during CAPD: the effect of a single dialysis cycle. *Clin. Sci.*, **65**, 539-545
49. Lindholm, B., Bergstrom, J. (1986). Nutritional aspects of CAPD. In Gokal, R. (ed) *Continuous Ambulatory Peritoneal Dialysis*, pp. 228-264. (Edinburgh: Churchill Livingstone)
50. Gokal, R., Ramos, J. M., McGurk, J. G., Ward, M. K., Kerr, D. N. S. (1981). Hyperlipidaemia in patients on CAPD. In Gahl, G., Kessel, M., Nolph, K. (eds) *Advances in Peritoneal Dialysis*, pp. 430-433. (Amsterdam: Excerpta Medica)
51. Ruben, J., Kirchner, K., Barnes, T., Teal, N., Ray, R., Bower, J. (1983). Evaluation of CAPD. *Am. J. Kidney. Dis.*, **3**, 199-204
52. Brown-Cartwright, D., Smith, H. J., Feldman, M. (1987). Delayed gastric emptying a common problem in patients on CAPD. *Perit. Dial. Bull.*, (Suppl) **7**, 510
53. Dulaney, J. T., Hatch, F. E. (1984). Peritoneal dialysis and loss of proteins. A review. *Kidney Int.*, **26**, 253-262
54. Kaysin, G. A., Schoenfield, P. Y. (1984). Albumin homeostasis in patients undergoing CAPD. *Kidney Int.*, **25**, 107-114
55. Bergstrom, J., Lindholm, B., Alverstrand, A., Hultman, E. (1985). Muscle composition in CAPD patients. In Greca, G. *et al.* (eds) *Proceedings 2nd International Course in Peritoneal Dialysis*, pp. 107-110. (Milan: Wichtig Editore)
56. Blumenkrantz, M. J., Kopple, J. D., Moran, K., Grodstan, G., Coburn, J. (1981). Nitrogen and urea metabolism during CAPD. *Kidney Int.*, **20**, 78-82
57. Mion, C., Slingeneyer, A., Canand, D. (1986). Peritonitis. In Gokal, R. (ed) *Continuous Ambulatory Peritoneal Dialysis*, pp. 163-217. (Edinburgh: Churchill Livingstone)
58. Gray, E. D., Peters, G., Verstagen, M., Regelman, W. E. (1984). Effect of extracellular slime substance from *Staph. epidermidis* on human cellular immune response. *Lancet*, **1**, 365-7
59. Dasgupta, M. K., Ulan, R. A., Bettcher, K. B. (1986). Effect of exit site infection and peritonitis on the distribution of biofilm encased adherent bacterial microcolonies on Tenckhoff catheters in patients undergoing CAPD. In Khanna, R. *et al.* (eds) *Advances in CAPD*, pp. 102-109. (Toronto: Univ. of Toronto Press)
60. Sombolos, K., Vas, S., Rifkin, O., Aylomainitis, A., McNamee, P., Oreopoulos, D. G. (1986). Propionibacteria isolates and asymptomatic infection of the peritoneal effluent in CAPD patients. *Nephrol. Dial. Transplant.*, **1**, 175-178
61. Van Bronswijk, H., Beelan, R. H., Verburgh, H. A. (1986). Recurrent peritonitis in CAPD. Survival and growth of bacteria within human mononuclear phagocytes. *Nephrol. Dial. Transplant.*, **1**, 113
62. Goldstein, C. S., Bomalaski, J. S., Zurrier, R. B., Neilson, E. G., Douglas, S. D.

(1984). Analysis of peritoneal macrophages in CAPD patients. *Kidney Int.*, **26,** 733–740

63. Keane, U. F., Comty, O. M., Verburgh, H. A., Peterson, P. K. (1984). Opsonic deficiency of peritoneal dialysis effluent in CAPD. *Kidney Int.*, **25,** 539–543
64. Lamperi, S., Carozzi, S. (1987). Interferons, peritoneal macrophages and peritonitis in CAPS patients. *Perit. Dial. Bull.* (Suppl) **7,** 546
65. Lamperi, S., Carozzi, S., Nasimi, M. G. (1986). Intraperitoneal immunoglobulin treatment in prophylaxis of bacterial peritonitis in CAPD. In Khanna, R. *et al.* (eds) *Advances in CAPD*, pp. 110–113. (Toronto: Univ. of Toronto Press)
66. Ballardie, F. W., Barsham, S., Clutterback, E. J., Brenchley, P., Bagston, R. (1987). IgG antibodies to coagulase-negative staphylococci in CAPD peritonitis: detection and role as potential opsonins. In Khanna, R. *et al.* (eds) *Advances in CAPD*, (Toronto: Univ. of Toronto Press) pp. 130–137
67. Randerson, D. H., Farrell, P. C. (1981). Long-term clearance variations in CAPD. In Atkins, R. C., Thomson, N., Farrell, P. C. (eds) *Peritoneal Dialysis*, pp. 27–28. (Edinburgh: Churchill Livingstone)
68. Slingeneyer, A., Canaud, B., Mion, C. (1983). Permanent loss of ultrafiltration capacity of the peritoneum and long-term peritoneal dialysis: an epidemiological study. *Nephron,* **33,** 133–138
69. Slingenyer, A., Elie, M., Mion, C. (1986). Sclerosing encapsulating peritonitis. Results of an international survey. *Nephrol. Dial. Transplant.,* **1,** 112
70. Shaldon, S. (1986). Peritoneal macrophage – the first line of defence. In Greca, G. *et al.* (eds) *Proceedings 2nd International Course on Peritoneal Dialysis*, pp. 201–204. (Milan: Wichtig Editore)
71. Nolph, K. D., Ryan, L., Moore, H. *et al.* (1984). A survey of ultrafiltration in CAPD. An international co-operative study – 2nd report. *Perit. Dial. Bull.,* **4,** 137–140
72. Verger, C. (1986). Clinical significance of ultrafiltration alterations on CAPD. In Greca, G. *et al.* (eds) *Proceedings 2nd International Course on Peritoneal Dialysis*, pp. 91–94. (Milan: Wichtig Editore)
73. Verger, C., Celicont, B. (1985). Peritoneal permeability and encapsulating peritonitis. *Lancet,* **1,** 486–487
74. Dobbie, J., Henderson, J., Wilson, L. (1987). New evidence of the pathogenesis of sclerosing encapsulating peritonitis obtained from serial peritoneal biopsies. *Perit. Dial. Bull.,* **6,** (Suppl) S5
75. Ota, K., Mineshima, M., Watanabe, N., Naganuma, S. (1987). Functional deterioration of the peritoneum: Does it occur in the absence of peritonitis. *Nephrol. Dial. Transplant.,* **2,** 30–33
76. Lamperi, S., Carozzi, S. (1987). Calcium antagonists improve ultrafiltration in CAPD patients. *Perit. Dial. Bull.,* (Suppl) **7,** 546
77. Coles, G. A. (1985). Is peritoneal dialysis a good long-term treatment? *Br. Med. J.,* **290,** 1164–1166
78. Broyer, M., Brunner, F. P., Brynger, H., Donckerwolcke, R. A., Jacobs, C., Kramer, P., Selwood, N. H., Wing, A.J. (1982). Combined report on regular dialysis and transplantation in Europe 1981. *Proc. Eur. Dial. Transplant. Ass.,* **19,** 4–59
79. Report of the national CAPD Registry of the National Institutes of Health 1986. Characteristics of participants and selected outcomes measures for the period January 1981 to December 1986. Publication of the national CAPD Registry of

the National Institute of Arthritis, Diabetes and Digestion and Kidney Disease, January 1987

80. Canadian Renal Failure Register 1985 report. Published by Kidney Foundation of Canada

81. Gokal, R., Jakubowski, C., Hunt, L., Bogle, S., Baillod, R., Marsh, F. P., Ogg, C., Oliver, D., Ward, M., Wilkinson, R. (1987). Multicentre study in outcome of CAPD and HD patients. *Lancet*, **2,** 1105–1109

82. Ataman, R., Burton, P., Walls, J., Brown, C., Gokal, R., Marsh, F. P. (1987). Long term CAPD: Some UK experience. *Perit. Dial. Bull.*, (Suppl) **7,** 52

83. Burton, P. R., Walls, J. (1987). Selection adjusted comparison of life-expectancy of patients on CAPD, haemodialysis and renal transplantation. *Lancet*, **1,** 1115–1119

84. Gokal, R. (1986). Worldwide experience, cost effectiveness and future of CAPD – its role in renal replacement therapy. In Gokal, R. (ed.) *Continuous Ambulatory Peritoneal Dialysis*, pp. 349–369. (Edinburgh: Churchill Livingstone)

85. Evans, R. W., Manminen, D. L., Garison, L. D., Hart, L. G., Blagg, C., Gutman, R., Hull, A. R., Lowne, E. G. (1985). The quality of life of patients with end-stage renal disease. *N. Engl. J. Med.*, **312,** 553–559

86. Stout, J., Gokal, R., Hillier, V., Kinsey, J., Auer, J., Oliver, D., Simon, G. (1987). The quality of life of high risk and elderly dialysis patients. *Dial. Transplant.*, **16,** 674–677

87. Fragola, J., Grube, J., VonBlock, L., Bourke, E. (1983). Multicentre study of physical activity and employment status on CAPD patients in the USA. *Proc. Eur. Dial. Transplant. Ass.*, **20,** 243–47

2
PERITONITIS COMPLICATING CAPD

A.J. BINT AND S.J. PEDLER

INTRODUCTION

Continuous ambulatory peritoneal dialysis (CAPD) is now established as a major modality for the management of chronic renal failure[1]. It has proved suitable as a medium-term treatment for the majority of patients, and as a long-term treatment for those patients for whom haemodialysis is either impracticable or contra-indicated including the young, elderly and those with diabetes mellitus.

In 1985 an estimated 27 000 patients worldwide were being managed by CAPD with 2450 of these in the UK. The major complication of CAPD is peritonitis[2,3]. Patients can expect on average one episode yearly although the incidence varies from centre to centre. However, many patients on treatment for much longer periods have never experienced this complication. Whilst most episodes of peritonitis can be managed successfully without disruption of peritoneal dialysis, infection can lead to temporary or permanent interruption of peritoneal dialysis as a result of changes in the peritoneal membrane or by the complete loss of the peritoneal cavity through adhesion formation, whilst occasional infections may prove fatal[4].

Since CAPD was first introduced, methods for the laboratory diagnosis and isolation of causal organisms continue to evolve. Moreover, agreement on the choice of appropriate antibiotics, their dosage, duration and route of administration is still lacking. It is our purpose, therefore, to discuss the diagnosis and management of CAPD-associated peritonitis.

PERITONITIS

Peritonitis during CAPD is defined by the presence of a cloudy peritoneal effluent associated with more than 100 white blood cells (WBC)/μl, and usually organisms in the dialysate effluent demonstrated either by Gram stain or culture. It is generally associated with clinical signs and symptoms of peritonitis[5] (Table 2.1).

Any degree of turbidity of the fluid should be regarded as of potential significance. However, cholecystitis, appendicitis, diverticular disease, pancreatitis and genito-urinary infection may all cause an increased white cell count in the effluent, with or without a positive culture[6]. Turbidity can also result from the presence of red blood cells in the effluent due to menstruation, ovulation, trauma or spontaneous bleeding. Occasionally, chyle and fibrinous material can lead to a turbid dialysate.

There may occasionally be less than 100 WBC/μl in cases of peritonitis and conversely a higher number when clinical peritonitis is absent[7]. Early morning effluent, because of the longer dwell time, is likely to have a higher white cell count. In bacterial peritonitis there is usually a preponderance of neutrophils. The rate of positive cultures in cases of clinical peritonitis should approach 90%. In units where

TABLE 2.1 Signs and symptoms of peritonitis in CAPD patients at presentation (modified from Prowant and Nolph[6])

	%
Cloudy dialysate effluent	97
Symptoms	
Abdominal pain	80
Nausea/vomiting	12
Chills	12
Diarrhoea	7
Signs	
Fever	29
Abdominal tenderness	76
Rebound tenderness	62
Drainage problems	15

the rate is less than 80% microbiological methods should be reviewed.

A relapse is a recurrence of peritonitis caused by the same organism following a course of treatment. This generally occurs within 7–14 days but may be a later event. It may be important to type organisms to indicate whether they are similar or not, as the recognition of relapsing infection will suggest catheter colonization, tunnel infection or intra-abdominal loculation of infection and will influence further management.

Clinical peritonitis usually occurs 24–48 hours after an episode of contamination at the time of an exchange. Other possible sources of infection include upper respiratory tract secretions and possibly transmural spread of organisms across the bowel wall. The average patient on CAPD using four exchanges daily will break the sealed system almost 1500 times per year. As Parsons et al.[8] commented, one error per year leading to peritonitis represents only 0.07% of the total exchanges and few, if any, patients can maintain this level of efficiency. Considering the number of skin scales carrying bacteria that are constantly shed and their attraction to plastic by electrostatic forces[9], it is perhaps surprising that peritonitis does not occur even more frequently. Host defence mechanisms, as well as scrupulous technique, may influence the individual patient's susceptibility to peritonitis.

MICROBIAL AETIOLOGY

The variety and frequency with which different organisms are isolated from episodes of peritonitis complicating CAPD are summarized in Table 2.2. This is based on a synthesis of published information from various centres and, although laboratory processing techniques varied, the pattern of infecting organisms is remarkably similar[2,10–13].

Staphylococcus epidermidis is responsible for almost half of the episodes of confirmed peritonitis. Other 'skin' organisms such as alpha-haemolytic streptococci, diphtheroids and *S. aureus* stress the importance of this site as a source of infecting organisms. The Enterobacteriaceae and *Pseudomonas aeruginosa* together account for almost a fifth of the infecting organisms and this has implications in the selection of initial empirical antimicrobial chemotherapy. Although fungal peritonitis is uncommon and generally caused by *Candida* spp.

TABLE 2.2 Organisms causing peritonitis in CAPD (compiled from Refs. 2, 10–13)

Organism	Mean percentage of total organisms isolated (range)	
Gram-positive bacteria		
Coagulase-negative staphylococci	41	(30–50)
Staphylococcus aureus	16	(7–24)
Viridans streptococci	9	(5–13)
Streptococcus faecalis	4	(2–11)
Diphtheroids	2	(0–7)
Gram-negative bacteria		
Escherichia coli	8	(1–14)
Pseudomonas aeruginosa	5	(0–8)
Klebsiella species	2	(1–6)
Other Gram-negatives	13	(7–21)
Anaerobic bacteria	< 2	
Fungi	2	
Mycobacteria	< 1	
Culture-negative	10–20	

it poses a particularly challenging management problem.

Among the miscellaneous organisms are included *Haemophilus influenzae*, *Bacillus* spp., *Pasteurella multocida*, *Serratia marcescens*, *Flavobacterium* spp., *Citrobacter* spp., *Alkaligenes* spp. and *Proteus* spp. It should be noted that anaerobic bacteria were rarely isolated in the series reviewed despite appropriate culture techniques. The isolation of anaerobes strongly suggests bowel perforation. *Mycobacterium* spp. are an extremely uncommon cause of infection but should be kept in mind in unresponsive infections. In a few episodes no pathogen can be isolated and this may either represent the presence of fastidious organisms or the presence of counts too low for detection.

DIAGNOSTIC PROCEDURES

Cell count

This confirms that turbidity of the effluent is due to increased white cells. A cell count in the effluent should be performed using a counting chamber, enumerating polymorphs and lymphocytes. In certain circumstances, for example culture-negative peritonitis, full differential staining should be performed. Excess numbers of eosinophils indicate eosinophilic peritonitis. Serial cell counts during therapy may be helpful in monitoring the therapeutic response[7].

Gram stain

A Gram stain of the centrifuged effluent deposit is likely to be positive in less than 30% of episodes of peritonitis[7,13,14]. Nevertheless, its simplicity and possible immediate value in determining whether a Gram-positive or Gram-negative pathogen or some unusual organism (e.g. a fungus) is present, make it a worthwhile procedure.

Culture

The concentration of bacteria in CAPD peritonitis may be lower than 1 colony forming unit/ml so that direct plating of uncentrifuged effluent is relatively insensitive[7]. It should not, therefore, be used as the sole method of culture. Sensitivity can be increased by centrifugation, filtration, broth culture of effluent, or a pour plate method[12,13]. It is very important that samples of effluent collected for bacteriological studies are not contaminated with bacteria from the skin of the patient or attendant. This may lead to misleading false-positive culture. Samples must therefore be collected with sterile precautions. We recommend that either the wall or a port of the bag is disinfected with alcohol and a 30 ml sample collected through this area with a needle and syringe. A 20 ml sample of this fluid should either be centrifuged and the deposit cultured and stained by Gram's method, or filtered through a bacteriological filter. Halves of the filter can be placed directly on two blood agar plates. Aerobic and anaerobic plates should be incubated for up to 72 hours. If the effluent is very cloudy, with fibrinous clots, centrifugation is preferable since filters often block.

Since even these methods may fail to detect very small numbers of bacteria, particularly fastidious pathogens such as anaerobes, we recommend that, in addition, 10 ml of effluent should be injected into aerobic and anaerobic blood culture bottles. These should be subcultured as soon as visible growth occurs or routinely at 48 hours and seven days, plates being incubated aerobically and anaerobically. This method has been shown to yield the highest percentage of positive cultures[13] but has the disadvantage that a viable count of bacteria in the fluid, which may be useful in following the course of therapy, cannot be obtained. Contamination with extraneous bacteria may lead to false-positive results. We believe, therefore, that this method should not be used alone. A flow chart of diagnostic methods is given in Figure 2.1.

If a bag cannot be cultured immediately, it should be refrigerated overnight at 4–8°C. It is essential that there is good cooperation between nephrology and microbiology departments to ensure that bags are handled and sampled in the most appropriate manner. We

FIGURE 2.1 Flow-chart of diagnostic procedures

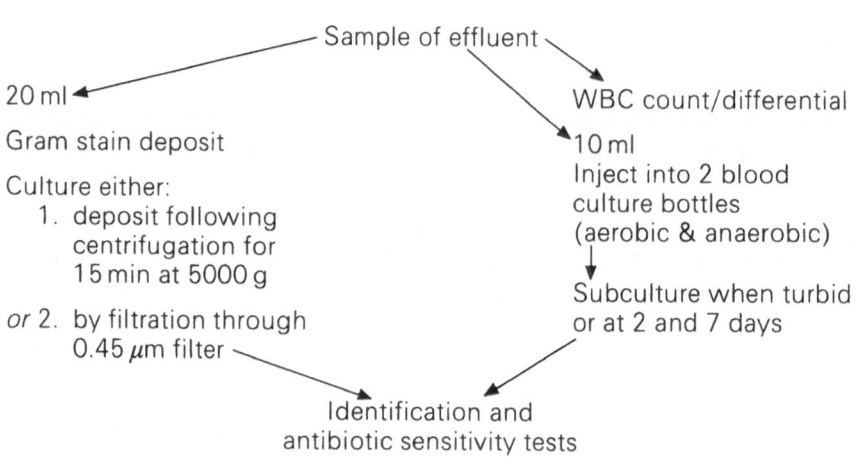

20 ml

Gram stain deposit

Culture either:
1. deposit following centrifugation for 15 min at 5000 g

or 2. by filtration through 0.45 μm filter

Sample of effluent

WBC count/differential

10 ml
Inject into 2 blood culture bottles (aerobic & anaerobic)

Subculture when turbid or at 2 and 7 days

Identification and antibiotic sensitivity tests

Incubate all plates at 35–37°C for up to 72 hrs, in air and anaerobically, with increased CO_2

do not believe that it is worthwhile culturing clear effluents on a routine basis, since occasional positive cultures do not necessarily predict impending peritonitis[7]. Neither should routine samples be cultured from patients on antibiotic treatment for peritonitis. However, should the effluent remain cloudy after 48–72 hours of treatment or the clinical circumstances warrant it, all diagnostic procedures should be repeated.

Routine blood cultures in cases of peritonitis are not worthwhile because they are rarely positive. However, if a patient is severely ill, toxic or shocked then blood cultures should be collected.

THERAPY

When peritonitis occurs in CAPD patients, prompt administration of appropriate antibiotics is essential. The infection then usually remains confined to the peritoneal cavity and rapid resolution will maintain the peritoneum as an efficient dialysing membrane. It is important that patients are trained to contact their renal units should the features of peritonitis occur.

We believe that intraperitoneal (ip) antibiotic administration is currently the best method of therapy. Precise concentrations of antibiotics designed to be therapeutic and non-toxic can be delivered directly to the site of infection. Intravenous therapy is usually unnecessary because bacteraemia is rare and for many antibiotics given ip adequate serum levels are obtained after a few hours[15,16]. However, in a particularly ill patient, an iv or ip loading dose can be given to ensure a faster rise in serum levels. Despite the attractions of ease of administration, reduced cost and elimination of manipulating the infusion system for drug addition, the efficacy of oral antibiotics alone is as yet unproven[13,17]. Most oral agents do not provide broad enough cover for initial therapy whilst gastrointestinal absorption may be particularly poor in patients with severe peritonitis. Oral drugs, however, may be suitable for continuation after initial ip therapy. A satisfactory first-line regime should cure about 80% of episodes without catheter removal and a further 10% should be cured by a further course of antibiotics without catheter removal. These criteria have not been satisfied by oral therapy alone to date.

We believe that continuation of CAPD with antibiotics added to the dialysis fluid is preferable to rapid cycling peritoneal dialysis. However, when patients are toxic or in severe pain, we recommend four no-dwell exchanges (lavage) with added antibiotics. Continuation of CAPD is easier and cheaper since less PD fluid and antibiotics are required and allows home treatment of peritonitis.

It is also common practice and probably useful to add heparin (500 U/L) to PD fluid in the presence of peritonitis to prevent fibrinous adhesions in the peritoneal cavity. We are not aware of any evidence other than anecdotal of the efficacy of this approach. It is also useful to increase the number of exchanges per 24 hours to five or six over the first two days, since with peritonitis there is a temporary decline in ultrafiltration and prolonged dwell periods could lead to fluid retention.

Any antibiotic regime designed for the immediate therapy of peritonitis must cover a large proportion of the usual pathogens (see Table 2.1). It is clear that an agent or combination of agents to cover both Gram-positive and Gram-negative pathogens is needed. However, local variations in frequencies of pathogen and antibiotic resistances may be important in determining antibiotic choice.

Data concerning stability of antibiotics, recommended ip doses and potentially toxic concentrations are given in Table 2.3, which contains information from many published papers[16,18-25], personal experiences, unpublished observations and manufacturer's data. In many instances different dose regimens for some antibiotics have been reported in the literature. We have tried to take into account known pharmacological data in CAPD patients. As far as stability of antibiotics in dialysis fluid is concerned most antibiotics are quite stable for up to 24 hours. However, since one cannot rule out some degree of instability, the problem can easily be avoided by adding the antibiotics to the bags immediately before use.

TABLE 2.3 Antibiotics useful in treating peritonitis in CAPD

Antibiotic	Loading dose iv or ip (mg)	Maintenance dose ip (mg/l)	Stability in dialysis fluid at room temperature (h)	Approximate maximum safe blood level (mg/l)	Comment
Penicillins					
Ampicillin	1000	125	48	300	
Cloxacillin	1000	125	24	300	
Ticarcillin	2000	250	24	300	
Azlocillin	2000	250	48	300	
Aminoglycosides					
Gentamicin	1.7 mg/kg	4–8	48	4 ⎫ Steady state Con-
Tobramycin	1.7 mg/kg	4–8	48	4 ⎪ sider alternate
Netilmicin	2.5 mg/kg	4–8	48	4 ⎬ bags or reduced
Amikacin	7.5 mg/kg	25	48	10 ⎪ dose Check blood
				⎭ level daily	
Cephalosporins					
Cefuroxime	750	125	24	100	
Cephalothin	1000	250	24	100	
Cefotaxime	1000	250	24	100	
Ceftazidime	1000	125	24	100	
Others					
Vancomycin	500	25	24	60–80	
Antifungal agents					
Amphotericin B	–	5	24	NK	Do not mix with antibiotics
Miconazole	–	20	NK	NK	
Flucytosine	–	50	NK	80	Check blood levels

NK, not known

ANTIBIOTICS

Aminoglycosides

These are the most problematic of the antibiotics to give by the ip route because of the risks of ototoxicity and nephrotoxicity, with loss of remaining renal function. If the widely-used dose of 8 mg/l is given in every bag, then after four or five days the serum level[16] reaches a plateau value of 4–5 mg/l. This is a potentially toxic level for gentamicin, tobramycin and netilmicin, and there are published instances of ototoxicity caused by gentamicin given at this dose[2]. Several regimens can reduce this problem at the price of added complexity. For example, after 48 hours the aminoglycoside can be given in alternate bags. This undoubtedly reduces the serum level, but at the risk of producing sub-therapeutic concentrations in the dialysis fluid for certain periods of time. Another option[14] is to reduce the dose to 4 mg/l after 48 hours treatment at the higher dose of 8 mg/l. We therefore recommend that if gentamicin is used, either of the regimens using drug-free bags or lower doses, after 48 hours should be used. We also recognize that tobramycin has been extensively used by some workers without overt clinical evidence of toxicity. Tobramycin and netilmicin are probably less toxic than gentamicin in humans[26,27]. An aminoglycoside blood level should be checked daily and for practical purposes this should not rise above 4 mg/l. An aminoglycoside should only be used for a maximum period of 7–10 days, provided that the isolate is sensitive and there is no suitable alternative agent. There is a need for carefully controlled comparative trials of these aminoglycosides in CAPD patients, with particular attention paid to incidence of toxicity.

Cephalosporins

Cefuroxime, cephalothin and cefamandole have all been used successfully in CAPD peritonitis. A significant advantage over the aminoglycosides is lack of toxicity in patients with renal failure. In the UK, cefuroxime has been a popular choice[2,19]. The cephalosporins mentioned are active against most Gram-positive bacteria, with the exception of *Streptococcus faecalis*, and many Gram-negative bacilli.

Strains of *Staph. epidermidis* should be tested in the laboratory with the cephalosporins; resistance cannot always be inferred from methicillin resistance[28-30]. Problems that have arisen in units using a cephalosporin as first-line therapy have included cases of pseudomembranous colitis[2], failures with resistant *S. epidermidis*[31], and infection with fungi. The third-generation cephalosporins such as cefotaxime and ceftazidime are more active than older cephalosporins against Gram-negative bacteria but less active against Gram-positive organisms. Ceftazidime includes activity against *P. aeruginosa*.

Penicillins

A number of penicillins are useful as ip agents for treating peritonitis. Ampicillin is the preferred agent for infections with *S. faecalis*. Cloxacillin can be used for staphylococcal infections. Antipseudomonal penicillins such as azlocillin or ticarcillin are indicated in *P. aeruginosa* infections in combination with an aminoglycoside[32].

Vancomycin

Vancomycin is a valuable drug for peritonitis caused by staphylococci and streptococci, particularly those strains resistant to other antibiotics. Fears concerning its toxicity have probably been over-stated in the past. Although potentially ototoxic, the recommended dose of 25 mg/L is well below the toxic levels of 60–80 mg/L[33]. For best-guess therapy it needs to be combined with an effective agent against Gram-negative bacteria such as an aminoglycoside[2] or a cephalosporin[34].

Practical antibiotic therapy

For the initial treatment of peritonitis on a 'best-guess' basis, a combination of vancomycin and an aminoglycoside would be satisfactory. This combination is preferable if unduly high resistance rates of *S. epidermidis* to cephalosporins are present[29]. Once the pathogen is known, either vancomycin or the aminoglycoside should be dis-

47

continued. Alternative initial regimes would be vancomycin plus a cephalosporin, or a cephalosporin alone.

S. epidermidis strains are particularly variable in their sensitivity pattern to antibiotics[29,30]. They are frequently resistant to methicillin, cloxacillin, cephalosporins and aminoglycosides. Fortunately, resistance to vancomycin is rare. Most Gram-negative bacilli in the UK, including *P. aeruginosa*, remain sensitive to gentamicin.

There is disagreement about the optimal length of treatment. A practical guide is to continue therapy for at least five days after the resolution of clinical signs and symptoms, and clearing of the effluent; usually 7–14 days is adequate[2,3,7]. Experience has not supported the need for more protracted therapy as used by some centres.

MISCELLANEOUS PROBLEMS

Culture-negative peritonitis

Although there was major debate about the aetiology of culture-negative peritonitis, the consensus points to this being caused by bacterial pathogens, the non-isolation reflecting inadequate microbiological culture techniques or inadvertent antibiotic usage by the patient before cultures are taken[35]. It should be possible to achieve an overall positive culture rate of $>90\%$ of all cases of peritonitis. Management of culture-negative cases is not different from culture-positive episodes as treatment will usually have been initiated. As usual, if there is no response after five to seven days then a full clinical and microbiological review is indicated, which will include a search for fastidious organisms.

Problem organisms

P. aeruginosa seems to produce a particularly aggressive and severe peritonitis[2,36]. The optimal therapy is an combination of an anti-pseudomonal penicillin (azlocillin or ticarcillin) and an aminoglycoside given ip[32]. An alternative agent is ceftazidime. *S. aureus* infections are usually more severe than those with *S. epidermidis* and have a tendency to abscess formation. This is sometimes heralded by the sudden appearance of cloudy fluid during or soon after a course of therapy. *Streptococcus faecalis* is resistant to cephalosporins and aminoglycosides though sensitive to vancomycin and ampicillin.

Persistent peritonitis

This implies peritonitis with a persistently cloudy effluent and positive culture unresponsive to appropriate therapy. Probable causes are catheter cuff and tunnel infection and ingrowth of bacteria into the catheter material[37]. These cases almost invariably require catheter removal followed by systemic antibiotics.

Perforation

Multiple organisms, especially Gram-negative aerobes and anaerobes, are strongly indicative of gut perforation. This complication is more prevalent in the elderly with diverticular disease and usually requires laparotomy and intensive systemic antibiotics although, occasionally, intensive lavage has led to a cure.

Fungal peritonitis

Although the incidence of this condition is low (1–2%) the morbidity and mortality are high[38]. Catheter removal is generally accepted as the most appropriate measure but ip therapy with antifungal agents without catheter removal has been successful[39]. Amphotericin B, flucytosine and miconazole have all been given ip. Oral therapy with ketoconazole alone is not advocated since poor absorption leads to low dialysate levels[40]. However, in combination with oral or ip flucytosine good results have been obtained without catheter removal[39].

49

Tuberculous peritonitis

The diagnosis of this condition is usually made at laparotomy for repeated attacks of peritonitis. Catheter removal is again essential together with appropriate antituberculous therapy[41]. It is unnecessary to give steroids.

Eosinophilic peritonitis

This does not constitute a major problem with an incidence of 2–4% of all episodes. It occurs soon after starting CAPD and is benign, asymptomatic, culture-negative and self-limiting[42]. Aetiological factors include 'allergy' to the materials and fluid used in the CAPD system and intraperitoneal blood. The use of steroids is only indicated if the eosinophilic response is prolonged and associated with severe symptoms[43].

Indications for catheter removal

These are catheter or tunnel infections, fungal, tuberculous and persistent peritonitis; bowel perforation; cuff erosion and protrusions; and post-transplant peritonitis. Catheter removal may also be indicated in cases of frequent repeated episodes of peritonitis. Antibiotics will need to be continued until there is clinical resolution. It is usually possible to reinsert the catheter 7 to 14 days later. With exit site infections related to the external subcutaneous dacron cuff, it is possible to exteriorize and shave off the cuff by a minor 'unroofing' surgical procedure. The tract, which is laid open, is allowed to granulate[44].

PREVENTION OF PERITONITIS

Proper facilities are required for running a CAPD programme. These include an adequate area for patient training and readmissions[45] staffed by an appropriate number of trained CAPD nurses (a nurse in charge plus an additional nurse for every 15 patients). When performing bag changes, patients should be taught a meticulous, aseptic technique, which should be standardized, consistent and well taught. Perfection of a bag exchange technique is the cornerstone of successful CAPD; however, with currently available systems, this is difficult to achieve although the aim must be to reduce accidental contamination. New types of connector devices may, in the next few years, minimize contamination-related peritonitis and early experience with ultraviolet and splice-sterile connecting devices appears promising. The use of in-line filters has been reported to reduce the incidence of peritonitis, though their role is not clearly determined as there are additional problems related to their use[46,47]. The Italian 'Y' connector double bag system, which works on the principle of drainage of dialysate fluid out of the peritoneum after the connections are made, is associated with a very low incidence of peritonitis (1 episode/53 patient months)[48]. This system is worthy of further extensive evaluation and use.

There is a lack of evidence to support long-term prophylactic antibiotic use[49]. However, after a known episode which might lead to contamination (e.g. unplanned disconnection), a single dose of ip cefuroxime (125 mg/l) or ip vancomycin (25 mg/l) is recommended.

REFERENCES

1. Gokal, R. (1986). World wide experience, cost effectiveness and future of CAPD – its role in renal replacement therapy. In Gokal, R. ed *Continuous Ambulatory Peritoneal Dialysis*, pp. 349–69. (Edinburgh: Churchill Livingstone)
2. Gokal, R., Ramos, J. M., Francis, D. M. A., *et al.* (1982). Peritonitis in continuous ambulatory peritoneal dialysis. Laboratory and clinical studies. *Lancet*, **2**, 1388–91
3. Editorial. (1982). Ambulatory peritonitis. *Lancet*, **1**, 1105
4. Fenton, S. S. A. (1983). Peritonitis-related deaths among CAPD patients. *Perit. Dial. Bull.*, **3** (Suppl), S9–S11
5. Pierratos, A. (1984). Peritoneal dialysis glossary. *Perit. Dial. Bull.*, **4**, 2–3
6. Prowant, B. F., Nolph, K. D. (1981). Clinical criteria for diagnosis of peritonitis. In Atkins, R. C., Thomson, N. M., Farrell, P. C., eds *Peritoneal Dialysis*, pp. 257–63. (Edinburgh: Churchill Livingstone)
7. Rubin, J., Rogers, W. A., Taylor, H. M., *et al.* (1980). Peritonitis during continuous ambulatory peritoneal dialysis. *Ann. Int. Med.*, **92**, 7–13
8. Parsons, F. M., Ahmed-Jushuf, I. H., Brownjohn, A. M., *et al.* (1983). CAPD peritonitis. *Lancet*, **1**, 348–49
9. Holmes, C. J., Allwood, M. C. (1977). The potential for contamination of intravenous infusion by airborne skin scales. *J. Hyg.*, **79**, 417–23

10. Slingeneyer, A., Mion, C., Beraud, J. J., Oules, R., Branger, B., Balmes, M. (1981). Peritonitis, a frequently lethal complication of intermittent and continuous ambulatory peritoneal dialysis. *Proc. Eur. Dial. Transplant Assoc.*, **18**, 212–21

11. Chan, M. K., Baillod, R. A., Chuah, P., *et al.* (1981). Three years' experience of continuous ambulatory peritoneal dialysis. *Lancet*, **1**, 1409–12

12. Fenton, P. (1982). Laboratory diagnosis of peritonitis in patients undergoing continuous ambulatory peritoneal dialysis. *J. Clin. Pathol.*, **35**, 1181–84

13. Knight, K. R., Polak, A., Crump, J., Maskell, R. (1982). Laboratory diagnosis and oral treatment of CAPD peritonitis. *Lancet*, **2**, 1301–04

14. Beardsworth, S. F., Goldsmith, H. J., Whitfield, E. (1983). CAPD peritonitis. *Lancet*, **1**, 348

15. Pancorbo, S., Comty, C. (1983). Pharmacokinetics of cefamandole in patients undergoing continuous ambulatory peritoneal dialysis. *Perit. Dial. Bull.*, **3**, 135–37

16. Paton, T. W., Manuel, A., Cohen, L. B., Walker, S. E. (1983). The disposition of cefazolin and tobramycin following intraperitoneal administration in patients on continuous ambulatory peritoneal dialysis. *Perit. Dial. Bull.*, **3**, 73–76

17. Johnson, C. A., Welling, P. G., Zimmerman, S. W. (1984). Pharmacokinetics of oral cephradine in continuous peritoneal dialysis patients. *Nephron*, **38**, 57–61

18. Neilson, H. E., Sorensen, I., Hansen, H. E. (1979). Peritoneal transport of vancomycin during peritoneal dialysis. *Nephron*, **24**, 247–77

19. Bint, A. J., Gokal, R. Paton, K. R., Sornes, S., Ward, M. K. (1980). Peritonitis in continuous ambulatory peritoneal dialysis: laboratory and clinical studies with cefuroxime. In *Cefuroxime Update: Royal Society of Medicine International Congress and Symposium Series No 38*, pp. 173–79. (London: Academic Press)

20. Local, F. K., Munro, A. J., Kerr, D. N. S., Sussman, M. (1981). Pharmacokinetics of intravenous and intraperitoneal cefuroxime in patients undergoing peritoneal dialysis. *Clin. Nephrol.*, **16**, 40–43

21. Oreopoulos, D. G., Williams, P., Khanna, R., Vas, S. (1981). Treatment of peritonitis. *Perit. Dial. Bull.*, **1**, (Suppl), S17–S19

22. Glew, R. H., Pavuk, R. A., Shuster, A., Alfred, H. J. (1982). Vancomycin pharmacokinetics in patients undergoing chronic intermittent peritoneal dialysis. *Int. J. Clin. Pharmacol. Ther. Toxicol.*, **20**, 559–63

23. Keogh, J. A. B., Carr, M. E., Falkiner, F. R., Martin, P., Grant, G., Keane, C. T. (1983). Pharmacokinetics of netilmicin in CAPD patients. *Perit. Dial. Bull.*, **3**, 172–75

24. Manuel, M. A., Paton, T. W., Cornish, W. R. (1983). Drugs and peritoneal dialysis. *Perit. Dial. Bull.*, **3**, 117–25

25. Sewell, D. L., Golper, T. A., Brown, S. D., Nelson, E., Knower, M., Kimbrough, R. C. (1983). Stability of single and combination antimicrobial agents in various peritoneal dialysates in the presence of insulin and heparin. *Am. J. Kidney Dis.*, **3**, 209–12

26. Smith, C. R., Lipsky, J. J., Laskin, O. L., *et al.* (1980). Double-blind comparison of the nephrotoxicity and auditory toxicity of gentamicin and tobramycin. *N. Engl. J. Med.*, **302**, 1106–09

27. Lerner, A. M., Reyes, M. P., Cone, L. A., *et al.* (1983). Randomised, controlled trial of the comparative efficacy, auditory toxicity and nephrotoxicity of tobramycin and netilmicin. *Lancet*, **1**, 1123–26

28. Davies, A. J., Dyas, A. (1985). Antimicrobial susceptibility of *Staphylococcus epidermidis* and *Staph. aureus. J. Antimicrob. Chemother.*, **15**, 127–28
29. Richardson, J. F., Marples, R. R. (1982). Changing resistance to antimicrobial drugs, and resistance typing in clinically significant strains of *Staphylococcus epidermidis. J. Med. Microbiol.*, **15**, 475–84
30. Gruer, L. D., Bartlett, R., Ayliffe, G. A. F. (1984). Species identification and antibiotic sensitivity of coagulase-negative staphylococci from CAPD peritonitis. *J. Antimicrob. Chemother.*, **13**, 577–83
31. Atkins, R. C., Humphrey, T., Thomson, N., Hooke, D., Williamson, J., Davidson, A. (1981). Efficacy of treatment in CAPD peritonitis – the problem of staphylococcal antibiotic resistance. In Atkins, R. C., Thomson, N. M., Farrell, P. C., eds *Peritoneal Dialysis*, pp. 333–39. (Edinburgh: Churchill Livingstone)
32. Leung, A. C. T., Orange, G., Henderson, I. S., Sleigh, J. D. (1984). Successful use of combined intraperitoneal azlocillin and aminoglycoside in the treatment of dialysis associated *Pseudomonas* peritonitis. *Perit. Dial. Bull.*, **4**, 98–101
33. Garrod, L. P., Lambert, H. P., O'Grady, F. (1981). *Antibiotic and Chemotherapy*, 5th edn., pp. 234–36. (Edinburgh: Churchill Livingstone)
34. Gray, H. H., Goulding, S., Eykyn, S. J. (1985). Intraperitoneal vancomycin and ceftazidime in the treatment of CAPD peritonitis. *Clin. Nephrol.*, **23**, 81–84
35. Vas, S. I. (1982). Aetiology and diagnosis of peritonitis in peritoneal dialysis patients. In La Greca G., Biasiol, S., Ronco, C., eds *Peritoneal Dialysis*, pp. 319–68. Proceedings of the first international course on dialysis. Vicenza, Italy, 1982. (Milan: Wichtig Editore)
36. Krothapalali, R., Duffy, W. B., Lacke, C., *et al.* (1982). *Pseudomonas* peritonitis and continuous ambulatory peritoneal dialysis. *Arch. Intern. Med.*, **142**, 1862–63
37. Locci, R., Romagnoni, M., Boccari, M., *et al.* (1984). Massive colonisation of an indwelling catheter by *Penicillium pinophilum* without peritonitis. *Perit. Dial. Bull.*, **4**, 243–44
38. Fabris, A., Biasioli, S., Borin, D., *et al.* (1984). Fungal peritonitis in peritoneal dialysis: our experience and review of treatments. *Perit. Dial. Bull.*, **4**, 75–77
39. Slingeneyer, A., Larochi, B., Stec, F., Canaud, B., Beraud, J. J., Mion, C. (1988). Oral ketoconazole plus intraperitoneal 5-flucytosine as the sole treatment of fungal peritonitis. In Maaher, I. F., Winchester, J. F., eds *Frontiers in Peritoneal Dialysis*. (New York: Field and Rich) (in press)
40. McGuire, N. M., Port, F. D., Kauffman, C. A. (1984). Ketoconazole pharmacokinetics in continuous ambulatory peritoneal dialysis. *Perit. Dial. Bull.*, **4**, 199–201
41. Khana, R., Fenton, S. S., Caltran, D. C., *et al.* (1980). Tuberculous peritonitis in patients undergoing CAPD. *Perit. Dial. Bull.*, **1**, 10–12
42. Gokal, R., Ramos, J. M., Ward, M. K., Kerr, D. N. S. (1981). 'Eosinophilic' peritonitis in continuous ambulatory peritoneal dialysis (CAPD). *Clin. Nephrol.*, **15**, 328–30
43. Salgia, P., Manos, J., Gokal, R. (1984). Cutaneous manifestations heralding eosinophilic peritonitis. *Perit. Dial. Bull.*, **4**, 265
44. Andreoli, S. P., West, K. W., Grosfeld, J. C., Bergstem, J. M. (1984). A technique to eradicate tunnel infection without peritoneal dialysis catheter removal. *Perit. Dial. Bull.*, **4**, 156–58
45. Oreopoulos, D. G. (1979). Requirements for the organization of a continuous ambulatory peritoneal dialysis program. *Nephron*, **24**, 261–63

46. Slingeneyer, A., Mion, C. (1982). Peritonitis prevention in continuous ambulatory peritoneal dialysis: long-term efficacy of a bacteriological filter. *Proc. Eur. Dial. Transplant Assoc.*, **19,** 388–96

47. Ash, S. R., Horswell, R., Heeter, E. M., Bloch, R. (1983). Effect of the Peridex filter on peritonitis rates in a CAPD population. *Perit. Dial. Bull.*, **3,** 89–93

48. Maiorca, R., Cantaluppi, A., Cancarini, G. C., Scalamogna, A., Broccoli, R., Graziani, G., Brasa, S., Ponticelli, C. (1983). Prospective controlled trial of a Y-connector and disinfectant to prevent peritonitis in continuous ambulatory peritoneal dialysis. *Lancet,* **2,** 642–44

49. Vas, S. I., Low, D. E., Oreopoulos, D. G., *et al.* (1981). Antibiotic prophylaxis in CAPD patients. In Atkins, R. C., Thomson, N. M., Farrell, P. C. eds *Peritoneal Dialysis,* pp. 320–26. (Edinburgh: Churchill Livingstone)

3
CAPD AND THE DIABETIC PATIENT

C. T. FLYNN

INTRODUCTION

It is recognized in the USA that diabetes mellitus is the most common single cause of end stage renal disease (ESRD)[1]. At the time that this recognition emerged, continuous ambulatory peritoneal dialysis (CAPD) became established as an accepted form of treatment for ESRD patients, taking a place alongside haemodialysis and renal transplantation[2]. The degree to which ESRD patients are accepted for any form of treatment, and if so, by which modality, is a reflection of complex social, political and economic factors which vary worldwide. In no subgroup of patients has this been more evident than in the case of diabetic ESRD patients. Where the general acceptance of patients has been low, as in the UK, the acceptance of diabetics has been especially low. Where the acceptance has been high, as in the USA, the proportion of diabetics entering ESRD programmes has been steadily rising, and is reaching 45% of all new patients[3]. This account will concern itself with the diabetic ESRD patient who has been accepted for treatment by CAPD. The complex interactions between CAPD, uraemia and diabetes will be presented, taken partly from the author's personal experience.

CAPD

The basic concept of CAPD is that the dialysate solution is left in the peritoneal cavity for several hours before being drained. This is in distinct contrast to other forms of peritoneal dialysis where the dwell time conventionally is 20–30 minutes. Continuous cycling peritoneal dialysis (CCPD) is a technique which developed out of the CAPD concept, and in which the dwell time is 3–4 hours. The long dwell time used in CAPD compensates for the low clearance rates. This concept was developed by Popovich and Moncrief in Austin, Texas in 1976[4]. In their early work they were restricted to the use of solutions in glass bottles and this impaired the mobility of patients and was the cause of a high peritonitis rate[5]. Oreopoulos, working in Canada, was able to use plastic bags which, after the dialysate had been instilled into the peritoneal cavity, could be folded up and carried in the patient's pocket or a pouch until the dialysate was drained[6]. The sterile dialysate contains an electrolyte solution approximating to that of plasma with the exception that bicarbonate is replaced by lactate (or acetate) and it lacks potassium. The solutions are made hypertonic by the addition of anhydrous glucose. Because of the greatly expanded use of these sterile, commercially produced solutions much work has been done on all aspects of the technology. These include devices to assist in the mechanical exchange, use of alternative osmotic agents to glucose, changes in the electrolyte compositions and variation in volume size. In the experience drawn on here most patients used 2 L volumes with solutions containing 1.5%, 2.5% or 4.25% dextrose, the 2.5% dextrose being the most common. Most patients had permanent silastic Tenck-hoff peritoneal catheters which were straight and had two dacron cuffs for fixation. The peritoneal catheter was connected by a titanium adaptor to a wider bore silastic tube, which had at its end a titanium spike for insertion into the inflow port on the dialysate bag. By using silastic for the connecting tube combined with the durability of titanium, the tube and spike were not routinely changed, some lasting over four years.

During the long dwell time uraemic toxins diffuse into the peritoneal cavity. Water is drawn into the solution by osmosis, and electrolytes by osmotic drag and diffusion, thus forming a urine which is drained out periodically and a new dialysis solution instilled. This exchange is made three or four times a day on a 7 day basis and the dialysis is thus almost continuous.

Glucose is almost completely absorbed during the dwell time presenting a glucose load of approximately 30–80 g to the patient, depending on the glucose concentrations used. Peritoneal dialysis is thus a form of haemodialysis in which the dialyser consists of the blood vessels of the peritoneum and the surrounding peritoneal membrane. The membrane is, of course, biocompatible, an issue of some concern in haemodialysis. In addition it allows the passage of higher molecular weight solutes than do haemodialysis membranes[7]. The major drawbacks of CAPD, as with all forms of peritoneal dialysis, are that it is invasive and liable to produce complications such as peritonitis, pericatheter and exit site infections, herniae and intra-abdominal disasters such as bowel perforation and, possibly, pancreatitis. In addition, it may cause abdominal distension, which is distasteful to 'figure conscious' patients; obesity, which may be severe; and a variety of abdominal complaints ranging from fullness to loss of appetite and an increased susceptibility to nausea and vomiting. By its nature CAPD was intended to be home treatment usually performed by the patient and not requiring clinic visits more often than once a month. Most publications have not indicated the number of patients performing self-care and the number that require help. Dependence upon help in the diabetic patient usually implies a failure to rehabilitate.

THE URAEMIC DIABETIC

The pathogenesis of diabetic nephropathy and its natural history are being intensely investigated and there is at least one journal devoted solely to this topic. Most insight has been gained by the study of type I (insulin-dependent) diabetics in whom the timing of pathological events is more distinct and who usually have no other diseases in the early years of diabetes. Type II (non-insulin-dependent) diabetics may develop identical complications but progression may be blurred by obesity, hypertension and cardiovascular disease.

After the onset of diabetes the kidneys may enlarge and have an increased glomerular filtration rate. Increased excretion of albumin occurs but does not reach detectable proteinuria by dip stick techniques, so called microalbuminuria. The degree of microalbuminuria may correlate with the later development of nephropathy[8]. The increased glomerular filtration rate may obscure the presence of renal disease. Eventually, after a period of 15–20 years, renal functional deterioration is apparent and heavy proteinuria and development of a nephrotic syndrome occur almost always in association with hypertension. Retinopathy and neuropathy also now develop[9]. These complications of chronic diabetes may vary in severity both between and in individual patients. However, the majority of Type I diabetics who develop ESRD have significant retinopathy and 50% may be blind.

There are many features in common between chronic renal disease and the chronic complications of diabetes. These are listed in Table 3.1. Firstly, like most chronic renal diseases, there is the same tendency for diabetic nephropathy to progress to ESRD. Once deterioration has started, the progression is faster in diabetes than in most other chronic renal diseases. Hypertension is frequently present in both and undoubtedly hastens progression of renal disease[10]. Neuropathy is another common feature and in poorly-treated patients may have devastating consequences. In diabetes, there is abnormal glycosylation of proteins whilst in uraemia there is abnormal carbamylation of proteins. Both can lead to a wide variety of dysfunctions of protein metabolism. Uraemic lung has long been known and frequently occurs in uraemic diabetics, worsened by the presence of a nephrotic syndrome. Severe oedema, with or without pulmonary oedema, is one

TABLE 3.1 Similarities of chronic diabetes and chronic renal disease

Progression to ESRD
Hypertension
Neuropathy
Dysfunction of protein metabolism
Carbohydrate intolerance
Pulmonary oedema
Fluid overload
Hyperlipidaemia
Cardiomyopathy
Pericarditis
Immunological disorders

of the more common indications for dialysis in diabetic patients. Hyperlipidaemia is another common feature and may be a link between the high incidence of atherosclerosis in both. Cardiomyopathies occur in both uraemic and diabetic patients. Among other complications, this may cause marked postural hypotension which may be a problem after haemodialysis or on CAPD. In our experience, diabetic ESRD patients seem more prone to pericarditis during intercurrent illnesses than non-diabetic, but pericarditis is a feature of both groups. Finally, the immune response is depressed in uraemics and is altered in many diabetics.

From the above it is obvious that it is often difficult to decide whether a particular manifestation is diabetic or uraemic. However, it seems reasonable to suppose that the manifestations of the uraemic state may occur at lower levels of conventional indicators, such as the serum creatinine, than in non-diabetic patients. It is also possible, although unprovable, that uraemia itself worsens the complications of chronic diabetes. Treatment by dialysis may be indicated at lower levels of creatinine, and in this regard serum creatinine may actually become unhelpful in decision making, and undue reliance may cause serious delay in starting treatment. The decision to dialyse, and by what method, is only one aspect of a complex medical and social situation and must not be taken in isolation. Type I diabetics tend to be relatively young, often have serious marital and family problems, are trying to cope with blindness, loss of job, impotence and diabetic control, as well as the medical problems of hypertension, fluid overload and uraemic symptoms. Type II diabetics tend to be middle-aged, and not so sharply demarcated from the general dialysis population. They tend to have less family and work problems, but are still plagued by many difficulties. On the brighter side, many diabetics do have a positive attitude and are motivated. An aggressive approach is indicated in these patients. This calls for a team of primary care givers including a physician, nurses, social workers and dietician. Regular eye examinations and aggressive therapy by laser, vitrectomy and other operations should be arranged. Care of the feet by teaching and regular examination should be a high priority.

POTENTIAL ADVANTAGES OF CAPD FOR THE DIABETIC

The general advantages are self-care, a less restricted diet as regards fluid, salt and potassium intake, steady state homeostasis avoiding the fluctuations inherent with haemodialysis, improved blood pressure control and a lessened incidence of pulmonary oedema, and improved blood sugar control (see Table 3.2).

TABLE 3.2 Potential advantages of CAPD for the diabetic

Self-care
Less restricted diet
Steady state
Blood pressure control
Blood sugar control
Less pulmonary oedema
No av fistula

Some of these advantages have particular relevance to the diabetic patient. Hyperglycaemia, due to lack of control, is accompanied by hyperkalaemia, induces thirst and may lead to excessive weight gains between haemodialyses. The presence of autonomic neuropathy may cause cardiac instability so that haemodynamic fluctuations of haemodialysis can be more severe in diabetics. The creation of an arteriovenous fistula may lead to ischaemia and necessitate amputation. CAPD does not require an arteriovenous fistula (and one should not be created as a back-up). Finally, the use of intraperitoneal insulin to control the diabetic has some advantages, which will be discussed in more detail later.

POTENTIAL DISADVANTAGES OF CAPD FOR THE DIABETIC

Obviously, these include those common to all CAPD patients, namely peritonitis, catheter-associated infections, herniae, obesity, etc. that were referred to earlier. For the diabetic the additional disadvantages include the large glucose loads – a practice usually avoided in the treatment of diabetics; the known tendency of diabetics to infection and hence to the infective problem of CAPD; the obscuring of intra-

TABLE 3.3 Potential
disadvantages of CAPD for
the diabetic

Susceptibility to infection
Peritonitis
Catheter problems
Herniae
Obesity
Large glucose loads
Silent bowel perforation
Increased vomiting
Neuropathic weakness
Blindness

---

abdominal complications which is already a known problem in diabetic patients (silent perforation); an increase in the incidence and severity of nausea and vomiting; and potential difficulties with self-care due to neuropathy and blindness (see Table 3.3).

SELECTION OF CAPD FOR DIABETIC PATIENTS

First, an assessment of the potential advantages and disadvantages must be made by the physician taking into account the factors mentioned above. If the patient is apathetic or depressed, a realistic appraisal must be made as to whether these may respond to enthusiastic training in self-care CAPD. Enthusiasm on the part of the staff must be tempered by reality and the patient must not be forced into a situation that would almost certainly fail. In marginal cases a CAPD nurse experienced in training is the best judge. Account should be taken of the patient's record of compliance, hospitalizations and social circumstances. If the patient has made a good adaptation to diabetic complications then the choice between CAPD and haemodialysis can be made by discussing them with the patient and arranging for the patient to talk with patients who are being successfully treated by both techniques. Neuropathy affecting hand muscles has not usually affected the ability to perform CAPD and can be helped further by the use of mechanical assist devices. If the patient has impaired vision it is relatively easy to decide whether they can do CAPD from the way that the patient copes with the activities of daily life. If the patient cannot do self-care, then the attitude and support of the family must be carefully assessed. If they live a long way from the haemodialysis unit CAPD may be chosen, but unless the family strongly wishes to do CAPD it is probably unwise to proceed. Even when the patient can be trained for self-care, the importance of the family support cannot be overemphasized if the outcome is to be successful.

TRAINING THE DIABETIC IN CAPD

It is essential that the patient be trained by an experienced nurse in a private area and with as few interruptions as possible. The physician should ensure that these conditions exist. CAPD clinics are much interrupted by phone calls and the CAPD nurses often have other dialysis duties so that organization is required to achieve these ends. The social worker and dietician must also be allowed adequate private time with the patient.

It is not possible to go into the training in much technical detail. Separate programmes are needed for the blind, non-blind diabetic and non-diabetic patients, as their needs differ. Training in diabetes, insulin action, hypoglycaemia, hyperglycaemia, blood pressure regulation, fluid balance and dietary control are all necessary in addition to performing CAPD training, recognition of peritonitis, exit site care and administration of intraperitoneal insulin.

One somewhat surprising discovery was how little many of the patients really understood diabetes, the action of insulin, the recognition of hypoglycaemia and dietary care. In some cases the lack of knowledge coexisted with an obsession with diabetes and a feeling that the patient was an expert. It requires time and patience and good humour to get the patient to accept the necessary modification in their control of diabetes.

INTRAPERITONEAL INSULIN AND CAPD

The first report of the use of intraperitoneal insulin in a peritoneal dialysis patient was in 1971[11]. This was in a patient who was on intermittent peritoneal dialysis and it was not used in the intervals between dialyses. With CAPD it became possible, because of the continuous nature of the treatment, to use intraperitoneal insulin as the only method of insulin administration. The total daily requirement is a little higher than twice the amount administered systemically prior to CAPD. The peritoneal dialysis catheter is usually inserted surgically some three weeks before the commencement of CAPD, but this time may be varied according to the patient's needs. The patient is again hospitalized for the initiation of intraperitoneal insulin. Type I diabetics who are insulin-dependent are usually more sensitive to insulin that Type II diabetics who often require higher doses of insulin. Fortunately, this increased requirement is not associated with more frequent hypoglycaemia because of the reduced responsiveness to insulin. Using a 4.25% dextrose dialysate the peak glucose level tends to be higher than with a 2.5% dextrose but the blood sugar levels at 8 hours tend to be similar, so that the dosage difference is minimal. However, with a 1.5% dextrose there is a greater risk of hypoglycaemia and the dose of insulin has to be reduced. We have found that if the use of 1.5% dextrose is avoided then the ratio of morning, afternoon and evening doses is 1:0.8:0.5.

There has been debate over the extent to which insulin is absorbed by the plastic containers and the general consensus is that it is small and relatively constant[12]. Others have studied the sites of absorption of insulin to determine to what extent it may be passing to the systemic rather than the portal circulation[13]. Clinical experience has been that the insulin dosage (and presumably the absorption) remain constant over time. Consequently, the favoured hypothesis is that the majority of the insulin is absorbed via the portal vein and thus passes first to the liver as with endogenous insulin in a non-diabetic.

CAPD with intraperitoneal insulin can therefore be considered a form of artificial pancreas[14]. Peritonitis has not seemed to alter the absorption of insulin to any marked extent. The dietary intake of food continues to have a marked effect upon blood sugar levels and periods of reduced food intake are often associated with reduced insulin

63

needs. Cessation of intraperitoneal insulin, e.g. when a patient has a peritoneal dialysis catheter removed, may result in severe rebound hyperglycaemia. Hypoglycaemia is a rare problem and although it is often asymptomatic, probably because of autonomic neuropathy, should be avoided.

We no longer strive for excellent control but are satisfied by moderately good control, which avoids hypoglycaemia and severe hyperglycaemia and daily monitoring of blood sugar. Blood sugar levels and glycohaemoglobin are measured on a monthly basis. Insulin doses are adjusted only if the glycohaemoglobin is consistently over 10%. Several patients do monitor their own blood sugar and some are obsessive about it. We have not found any improvement in their blood sugar control than in patients with a more relaxed attitude. As one of the reasons for using intraperitoneal insulin is to avoid the necessity for subcutaneous insulin, repeated monitoring of blood sugar would seem to offer little benefit to a clinically stable patient whose glycohaemoglobin is acceptable. However, some patients will disagree with this as perhaps will a majority of physicians. We have one patient, our longest surviving diabetic on CAPD, who developed resistance to intraperitoneal insulin whilst maintaining sensitivity to systemic insulin, albeit in high dosages. It is presumed that the patient may have developed antibodies on the peritoneal membrane but this cannot be proved. The value of the glycosylated haemoglobin has not been fully substantiated in dialysis patients. Both the shortened red cell survival and carbamylation may affect the results. It has been suggested that glycosylated albumin might be better[15]. However, as judged by the blood sugar response to increased insulin given when the glycosylated haemoglobin was over 10%, it seems to be an acceptable marker of diabetic control.

BLINDNESS IN THE DIABETIC ON CAPD

As has been mentioned earlier it is relatively easy to determine whether a diabetic with impaired vision can successfully perform the CAPD exchange. Nevertheless, a selected patient will still require meticulous training. Aids for drawing up the insulin, measuring the dose and for injecting the insulin into the bag are necessary. Mechanical devices to help with the spike transfer are not usually necessary, but may serve to give the patient confidence. Blind patients take no longer than sighted patients to do the exchanges and do not feel any undue anxiety. Partially sighted patients may benefit from large print instruction and magnifying glasses. Such patients, however, do no better than totally blind patients. The lifestyle of each blind patient must be individually examined and an appraisal made of the support provided to them by family members. On this depends such mundane matters as storage of supplies, the correct identification of solutions of differing glucose concentrations, the selection of the correct dose of insulin and the recognition of peritonitis or the presence of blood in the bag.

PERITONITIS AND THE DIABETIC ON CAPD

In our experience patients were divided into non-diabetic, sighted diabetic and blind diabetic for the purpose of analysing peritonitis episodes. The peritonitis rates of all patients treated since 1978 can be seen in Table 3.4. Table 3.5 shows the rates for current patients. The peritonitis rates for current patients expressed as the number of weeks

TABLE 3.4 Peritonitis rates – all patients

Patients	CAPD days	Episodes of peritonitis	Weeks/episode of peritonitis
All non-diabetic	38 812	114	48.6
All sighted diabetic	9 981	42	33.9
All blind diabetic	25 996	82	45.3

TABLE 3.5 Peritonitis rates – current patients

Current patients	CAPD days	Episodes of peritonitis	Weeks/episode of peritonitis
Non-diabetic	15 092	23	93.7
Sighted diabetic	5 707	12	67.9
Blind diabetic	9 937	17	83.5

per incident of peritonitis compare favourably to those quoted in the NIH CAPD Registry in the USA and by the EDTA/ERA in Europe. The type of organism did not differ from that found by other CAPD clinics. *Staphylococcus epidermidis, S. aureus, Pseudomonas, E. coli*, miscellaneous and fungal organisms were found in descending order of frequency. The distribution of organisms was not different between diabetics and non-diabetics. Exit site infections were predominately *S. aureus* with *Pseudomonas* a much lower second. Fears that diabetics may suffer more infective complications on CAPD than non-diabetics were not confirmed.

METABOLIC PROBLEMS OF THE DIABETIC ON CAPD

Elevated lipid levels have long been known to occur in renal failure patients[16]. It has been reported that some patients transferred to CAPD were noted to have a worsening of any pre-existing hyper-triglyceridaemia[17]. The majority of Type I diabetics on intraperitoneal insulin had normal levels of cholesterol and triglycerides[18]. The exceptions to this were the patients who smoked cigarettes. Non-diabetic patients whose glucose tolerance deteriorated on CAPD developed hyperglycaemia, elevated glycohaemoglobins and elevated serum lipids. With the use of intraperitoneal insulin, fasting blood sugar was brought to normal and the glycohaemoglobin reduced to below 10% but in no case did the hypertriglyceridaemia improve, thus excluding intraperitoneal insulin as the reason for the normal lipid levels in most Type I diabetic patients on CAPD.

Serum albumin tended to be below normal range in the majority of patients on CAPD whether diabetic or not. Such levels invariably fell during an episode of peritonitis but usually improved after recovery. In such cases protein supplements were often used but were never very popular. Protein malnourishment did not correlate with either serum creatinine or haemoglobin levels.

BLOOD PRESSURE CONTROL OF DIABETICS ON CAPD

Very few diabetic patients on CAPD required antihypertensive therapy. Blood pressure is influenced by the intake of fluid and salt and several did become intermittently hypertensive when fluid and salt overloaded. Supine blood pressure was considerably higher than standing blood pressure in the majority of patients. Episodes of dehydration are often associated with quite severe postural hypotension which produces symptoms of weakness and nausea. This can be a relatively urgent situation and the dehydration should be corrected by a salty broth, by fluid as early as possible and not allowing the patient to become prostrate. This aspect receives considerable attention during the training of the patient.

NAUSEA AND VOMITING

Many diabetic patients have gastroparesis. This is associated with delay in gastric emptying and the presence of undigested food in the stomach long after it has been eaten. However, nausea and vomiting tend to occur in discrete episodes and respond rather rapidly to hospitalization and intravenous therapy. Diabetic patients on haemodialysis have similar episodes of nausea and vomiting which, although unpleasant, may actually be beneficial to a patient who consistently has large weight gains between dialyses or pre-dialysis hyperkalaemia. In the diabetic patient on CAPD who is continually losing considerable volumes of salt water, nausea and vomiting may quickly lead to dehydration which in turn causes weakness and nausea which, if prolonged more than two days, will lead to hospitalization. Treatment is by rehydration using intravenous therapy and limitation of oral intake to bland liquids or semiliquid foods. Intravenous cimetidine and metoclopramide are thought to be efficacious in speeding resolution of the problem but this cannot be scientifically proved. The curious thing is why with a fixed anatomical abnormality these episodes should be so intermittent in nature. Careful dietary analysis suggests that often the patient has indulged in meals that are entirely inappropriate and difficult to digest prior to the onset – after which the process becomes self-sustaining. There is also some suggestion that emotional stress,

67

possibly exacerbated by dietary non-compliance, can induce these episodes.

TERMINAL CARE OF DIABETICS ON CAPD

As described earlier, some patients may be placed on CAPD by the choice of a caring relative despite being unable to perform the exchange procedure. A few patients performing self-care CAPD have deteriorated to the point where a relative takes over the care, usually by gradual increments in the help given. In some cases the patient could probably have continued to do more but the relatives were overly concerned to take responsibility. Due to the gentle and continuous nature of CAPD, such patients probably survived longer than they would have done on haemodialysis. In such circumstances, the CAPD exchange was rarely the cause of any difficulty or distress to the caring relative. Most stress came simply from caring for a terminally ill patient; whether the prolongation of the phase is considered as good or bad is a matter for personal evaluation by the family and physician. Certainly the family needs a lot of support; the physician should make house calls if needed. Discontinuing treatment is an option but most families, at least in the USA, would be unwilling to take that responsibility at home.

PATIENT AND TECHNIQUE SURVIVAL OF DIABETIC PATIENTS ON CAPD

Actuarial analysis of survival both for patients and technique and for both combined have been made. The CAPD technique success analysis is shown in Figure 3.1. Technique success is defined as follows: any patient who is changed to haemodialysis is considered a technique failure – that is, another mode of treatment was chosen over CAPD. (No patient who was a primary candidate for transplantation was placed on CAPD in this series.)

The most important point is that technique survival is good in diabetic patients. Conversely, this means that diabetics will tend to stay on CAPD and not drop-out, primarily to haemodialysis. A

68

CAPD Technique Success
Through September 15, 1986

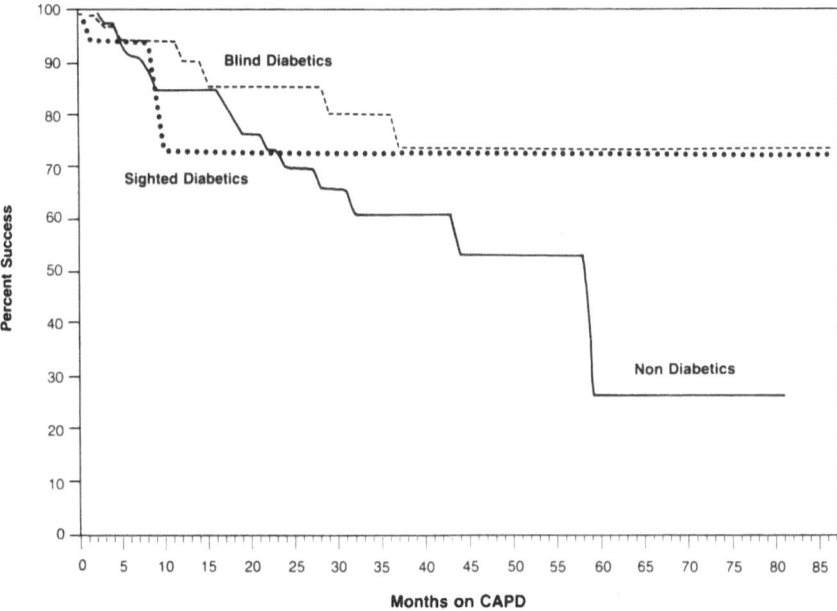

FIGURE 1.3. This shows the actuarial analysis of technique survival. A failure is defined as transfer to hemodialysis (no patients were transplanted). Death while on CAPD is not considered a technique failure

concern in the UK has been expressed that there are inadequate haemodialysis facilities and a high drop-out rate from CAPD. This might cause reluctance to place diabetics on CAPD, which does not seem justified.

CONCLUSION

CAPD has proved an effective treatment for diabetic patients with ESRD. Patient survival is acceptable and patient technique survival is better than in non-diabetics. Quality of life for self-care patients is superior to that on haemodialysis. The complications of CAPD *per se* are not greater among the diabetic than the non-diabetic patients. Intraperitoneal insulin is a useful and effective way of achieving diabetic control. Prolongation of the terminal phase of the life of a diabetic on CAPD is a matter for concern. Nausea and vomiting are more significant problems with patients on CAPD than on haemodialysis. Haemodialysis and renal transplantation should be available if the full potential for CAPD is to be realized.

ACKNOWLEDGEMENTS

I would like to thank all the CAPD nurses who cared with me for patients in the Nephrology Clinic and at Iowa Lutheran Hospital. I would also like to thank my Office Manager Kaye Clark and our word processing expert Brian Kirkpatrick for their hard work and enthusiastic support.

REFERENCES

1. Sergimoto, T., Rosansky, S.J. (1984). The incidence of treated end stage renal disease in the Eastern United States. *Amer. J. Public Health,* **74,** 14–17
2. Popovich, R.P., Moncrief, J.W., Nolph, K.D., Grode, A.J., Twardowski, Z.J., Pyle, W.K. (1978). Continuous ambulatory peritoneal dialysis. *Ann. Int. Med.,* **88,** 449–456
3. Freidman, E.A. (1986). Retinal history of diabetic nephopathy. In *Diabetic Nephropathy Strategy for Therapy,* **5,** 65–83. (Boston, MA: Martinus Nijhoff Publishing)
4. Popovich, R.P., Moncrief, J.W., Decherd, J.F. (1976). The definition of a novel, portable/wearable equilibrium peritoneal dialysis technique. *Am. Soc. Artif. Int. Org.* **5,** 64 (Abstr)
5. Moncrief, J.W., Popovich, R.P., Nolph, K.D. (1978). Additional experience with continuous ambulatory peritoneal dialysis (CAPD). *Trans. Am. Soc. Artif. Int. Org.,* **24,** 476–483
6. Oreopoulos, D.G., Clayton, S., Dombros, N., Zellerman, G., Katirtzoglou, A. (1979). Nineteen months experience with continuous ambulatory peritonal dialysis (CAPD). *Proc. Eur. Dial. Transplant Assoc.,* **16,** 178–183
7. Babb, A.L. Johansen, P.J., Straud, J.J., Tenckhoff, H. Simibner, B.H. (1973). Bidirectional permeability of the human peritoneum to middle molecules. *Proc. Eur. Dial. Transplant Assoc.,* **10,** 247–262
8. Mogensen, C.E. (1984). Editorial review: Microalbuminuria and incipient diabetic nephropathy. *Diabetic Nephropathy,* **3,** 75–78
9. Freidman, E.A. (1986). Natural history of diabetic nephropathy. In *Diabetic Nephropathy Strategy for Therapy,* **5,** 65–83. (Boston, MA: Martinus Nijhoff Publishing).
10. Mogensen, C.E. (1976). High blood pressure as a factor on the progression of

diabetic nephropathy. *Acta Med. Scand. Suppl.*, **602**, 29–32
11. Crosley, K., Kjellstrand, C. M. (1971). Intraperitoneal insulin for control of blood sugar in diabetic patients during peritoneal dialysis. *Br. Med. J.*, **1**, 269–270
12. Twardowksi, Z. J., Nolph, K. D., McGary, J., Moore, H. L. (1983). Influence of temperature and time on insulin absorption to plastic bags. *Am. J. Hosp. Pharm.*, **40**, 583–586
13. Schade, D. S., Eaton, R. P. (1980). The peritoneum – a potential insulin delivery route for a mechanical pancreas. *Diabetes Care*, **3**, 229–234
14. Flynn, C. T., Nanson, J. (1979). Intraperitoneal insulin with CAPD – an artificial pancreas. *Trans. Am. Soc. Artif. Int. Org.*, **25**, 114–116
15. Peterson, C. M. and Jovanovic, L. (1986). Insulin oral agents and monitoring techniques. In *Diabetic Nephropathy Strategy for Therapy*, 9–32 (Boston MA: Martinus Nijhoff Publishing)
16. Bagdade, J. D., Ponte, D. J., and Bierman, L. (1968). A metabolic consequence of chronic renal failure. *N. Engl. J. Med.*, **279**, 181
17. Amair, P., Klanna, R., Leibel, B., Pierratos, A., Vas, S., Meema, E., Blair, G., Chisholm, L., Vas, M., Zingg, W., Digenis, G., Oreopoulos, D. (1982). Continuous ambulatory peritoneal dialysis in diabetics with end stage renal disease. *N. Engl. J. Med.*, **306**, 625
18. Flynn, C. T. and Shadur, C. A. (1981). A comparison of continuous ambulatory peritoneal dialysis in diabetic and non-diabetic patients. *Am. J. Kidney Dis.*, **1**, 15–23

4

CAPD AND THE ELDERLY PATIENT

A. J. NICHOLLS

INTRODUCTION

The prevalence of end-stage renal disease (ESRD) increases rapidly with advancing age; Figure 4.1 shows that 50% of all patients presenting with ESRD are over 55 years old. In 1970 the average age of patients starting dialysis in Europe was 35 years[1] but recent reports from France and the USA have indicated a mean age of new patients of nearly 60 years[2,3], with 40% older than 60 years[4,5]. The elderly patient with ESRD has posed an increasing challenge to nephrologists in the past five years, with a variety of moral, medical and economic issues emerging.

Since its introduction in the late 1970s[6,7], CAPD has had enormous impact on the provision of ESRD services for patients of all ages. Many more patients have been treated at home but decisions about treatment strategies have not always been based upon published data[8]. Certainly CAPD has permitted dialysis in Britain for large numbers of elderly patients who had previously been denied treatment[9], but in other countries where haemodialysis facilities are not restricted (as they are in Britain) CAPD has emerged as the treatment of choice for the elderly patient[10]. It would appear, however, that medical decision-making about CAPD in the elderly has been intuitive rather than logical, with the widespread application of the technique resembling the typical 'honeymoon stage' of new technologies and drugs[11]. Rational assessment of new techniques often follows rather than precedes their widespread introduction: that has been true of CAPD

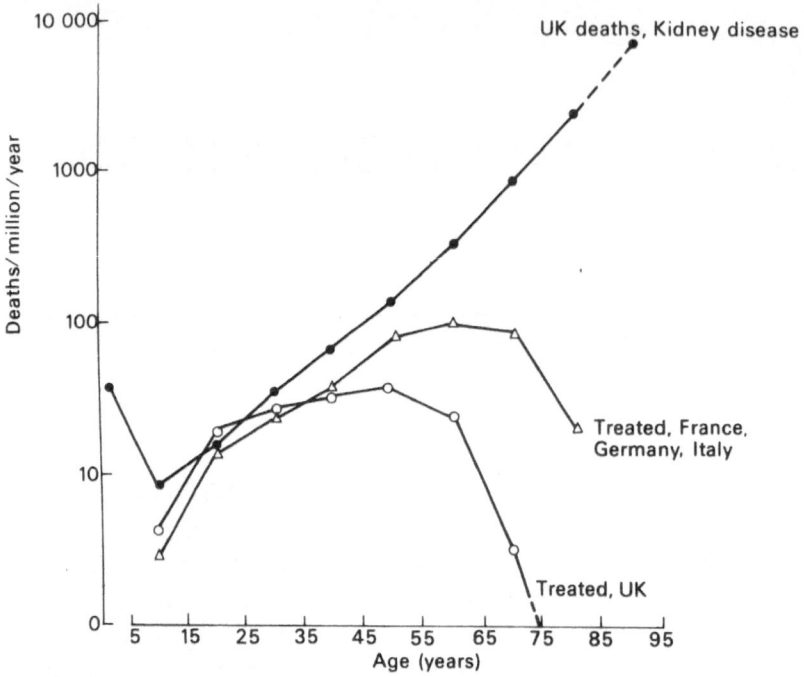

FIGURE 4.1   Age-specific rates for kidney disease in the United Kingdom with data for age-specific treatment rates for end-stage renal failure for France, Germany, Italy and the United Kingdom. Data from Registrar General UK 1976 and European Dialysis and Transplant Association. (Adapted from Cameron, S. (1981). *Kidney Disease: The Facts*, p. 160. (Oxford: Oxford University Press), with permission)

in the elderly as of any other medical innovation. This review concentrates on selection of elderly patients for CAPD, its technical aspects, the results of treatment and comparisons with both haemodialysis and other peritoneal dialysis strategies.

It must be stressed as a rider to this analysis that beyond a certain point comparisons between CAPD and haemodialysis are meaningless, rather like debating whether a bicycle or car is the 'better' means of transport. The car is quicker, the cycle cheaper; the car less energetic, the cycle healthier, but neither is universally to be preferred to the other. Likewise, the ESRD patient with several failed fistulae would regard CAPD as superior to haemodialysis, as a person with no driving licence would prefer a bicycle to a car: on the other hand the patient with no peritoneal cavity as a result of surgical adhesions would find choice between treatments equally redundant.

In essence then, it will be accepted that both CAPD and haemodialysis are viable treatments for some elderly patients, while neither is ideal for all patients. Very little attempt will be made to pursue an elusive universal 'gold standard' of dialysis treatment for the elderly, as the complexity of medical problems other than ESRD makes these patients so heterogeneous.

DEMOGRAPHY OF RENAL FAILURE IN THE ELDERLY

The age-specific incidence of ESRD rises with increasing age. The provision of renal replacement therapy varies widely from country to country and this disparity is most marked for the elderly patient[12] (Figure 4.2). For patients aged under 65 years, virtually all European countries have an acceptance rate between 30 and 50 patients per million population per year. On the other hand, in the over-65 age group the age-specific acceptance rate reaches nearly 100 per million population in Belgium and is over 70 in West Germany, Italy, Sweden and Switzerland; in East Germany virtually no patients over 65 receive renal replacement therapy and in Britain around 20 per million population are accepted annually for treatment.

If comprehensive renal replacement therapy is provided irrespective of the age of patients, however, one may expect at least 40% of all new patients to be aged over 60 at the start of treatment. As many of these patients are unsuitable for home haemodialysis, no treatment was available in countries like Britain, where hospital haemodialysis resources were limited, until the advent of CAPD. CAPD has thus allowed many patients to survive when no reasonable alternative form of therapy existed[9], but the tendency to treat elderly patients with CAPD rather than let them die has led to an almost universal and paradoxical acceptance of CAPD as the preferred mode of treatment for such patients, even when resources allow alternative treatment strategies. The next section will consider in more detail the selection of patients for CAPD, assuming that haemodialysis is available as an alternative treatment.

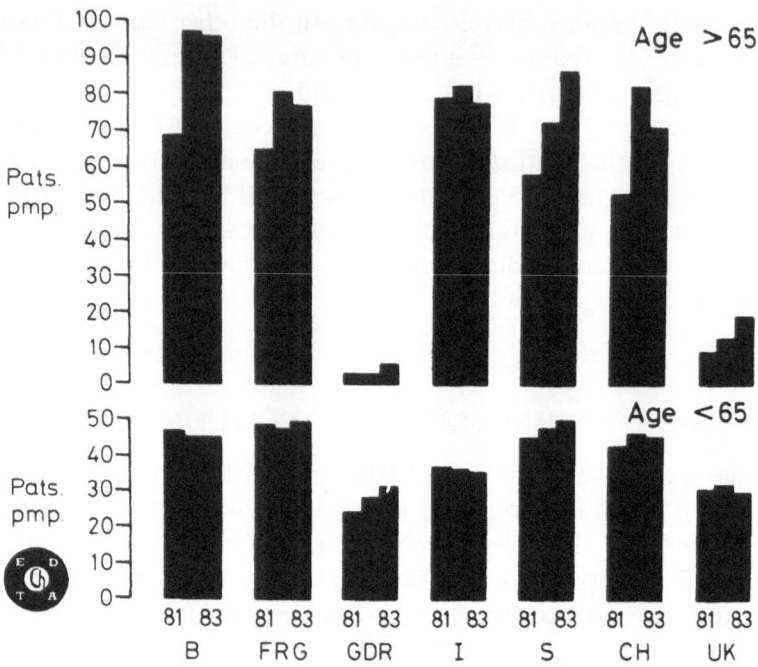

FIGURE 4.2 Age-specific acceptance rates per million population (PMP) for renal replacement therapy between 1981 and 1983 in Belgium (B), Federal Republic of Germany (FRG), German Democratic Republic (GDR), Italy (I), Sweden (S), Switzerland (CH), and the United Kingdom (UK). From EDTA Annual Report, 1984 (Ref. 11), with permission

SELECTION OF PATIENTS; INDICATIONS AND CONTRAINDICATIONS TO CAPD

Elderly patients with renal failure often have a variety of other medical problems which may dictate the preferred method of dialysis treatment. More than half of patients over the age of 60 will have clinical evidence of cardiovascular disease at the time of presentation with renal failure[14]. If they have suffered a previous myocardial infarction or have long-standing hypertension and/or atherosclerosis, haemodialysis is likely to be accompanied by symptomatic hypotension, cramps, or other distressing symptoms[15]. Such patients are, therefore,

76

best treated by CAPD provided they are motivated towards this form of treatment and have an adequate peritoneal cavity.

Many older patients develop uraemic symptoms requiring dialysis whilst still retaining a residual glomerular filtration rate (GFR) of 2 ml/min or more. The consequent urine output of a litre or more daily will ensure little weight gain between dialyses and so relatively trouble-free haemodialysis. If a usable arteriovenous fistula proves elusive, CAPD will be the only treatment option, but may be accepted as a semi-temporary measure until permanent vascular access can be established. An elective switch to haemodialysis need not in these circumstances be regarded as a CAPD treatment failure. Poor vision is not necessarily a contraindication to CAPD, but in elderly patients it may be associated with lack of manual dexterity and a lack of motivation. Training blind elderly patients for CAPD is thus not as successful as young blind diabetics, in whom outstanding results have been reported[16]. Arthritis of the fingers may make bag changing difficult but this can usually be overcome by means of commercially available connect/disconnect aids.

Although CAPD is often advocated as a suitable form of treatment for the single patient (and this is obviously more common in the elderly as a result of bereavement), social isolation often mitigates against successful long-term treatment[17]. Hence, although CAPD may free the unit of such patients who would otherwise be on hospital-based haemodialysis, it would be wrong to assume that it is necessarily ideal for them. Indeed, such socially isolated patients with renal failure often gain from the social interaction of thrice-weekly hospital haemodialysis sessions[18] and one may thereby expect their overall rehabilitation and life satisfaction to be greater. Results of CAPD are better when there is the support of a spouse or other close relative available for the patient, even though the technical aspects of the treatment itself are primarily the responsibility of the patient. Patients with depression or impaired cognitive function are unsuitable for CAPD and must be carefully assessed in this regard or else futile attempts could be made to train patients better treated by hospital haemodialysis.

As has been pointed out in the past, if CAPD is reserved for 'second class' patients (by virtue of age, complicating diseases, psychological state, social isolation, disability or lack of motivation) it is inevitable

TABLE 4.1   Relative indications for CAPD or haemodialysis in the elderly

CAPD	Haemodialysis
Clinical cardiovascular disease	Inadequate peritoneal function
Little residual renal function	Little motivation for self-care
No fistula	Poor vision
Desire to travel	Social isolation
Long distance from haemodialysis centre if home HD not feasible	Dislike of change in body image

that CAPD will be regarded as a second rate treatment[19]. Table 4.1 lists relative indications for CAPD in the elderly, compared with haemodialysis.

TECHNICAL ASPECTS

Catheter insertion

Insertion of a chronic peritoneal dialysis (PD) catheter under local anaesthesia using a trocar causes minimal upset to the patient, and is thus desirable for the older patient in whom the risks of general anaesthesia and laparotomy are increased. Nonetheless, the technique carries the penalty of several complications, the most serious of which are bowel puncture and intraperitoneal haemorrhage. Both these hazards are more likely when there are adhesions due to previous abdominal surgery and/or peritonitis, and hence pose a particular risk to elderly patients who commonly have a scarred abdomen. Previous abdominal surgery should generally be regarded as an indication for catheter insertion at laparotomy; in the unfit patient, use of the needlescope device[20] to identify adhesions may prove an advantage, but has not been extensively evaluated in older patients.

Catheter migration is infrequent in older patients, who tend to have a less active omentum; thus the use of either a straight or curled Tenckhoff catheter is acceptable. Alternative access devices such as the column-disc catheter[21] or Toronto Western Hospital catheter[22] are unnecessary. Furthermore, as both these devices require laparotomy for removal, they are best avoided in the elderly lest emergency removal is needed in the presence of intractable peritonitis.

As in younger patients, trocar insertion of a PD catheter is best performed after priming the abdomen with 2 L of heparinized dialysate via a plastic intravenous cannula or temporary PD catheter. The distended abdomen permits safe trocar insertion, while the fluid instilled allows an immediate check to be made on catheter placement and free drainage.

The elderly patient is particularly prone to constipation, so pre-insertion bowel clearance is essential to avoid pelvic displacement of the catheter. In males, bladder catheterization is often necessary before PD catheter insertion lest a chronically distended bladder be inadvertently punctured.

In a personal series of nearly 200 Tenchkoff catheter insertions under local anaesthesia using the technique and precautions outlined above, intra-abdominal haemorrhage requiring laparotomy has occurred only once, bladder puncture (which settled on catheter drainage) once, and there have been no instances of bowel perforation (personal data, unpublished). Thus, in the elderly patient the gain from avoiding laparotomy has been considerable, with minimal risks.

Patient training

Whenever possible, elective early PD catheter insertion will allow a period of 24 to 36 hours for catheter flushing with small volume (500 ml) fills immediately post-insertion, followed by a period of a week or so with no dialysis. This allows the patient home from hospital, thereby regaining mobility, regular bowel actions, and confidence, all of which are often lost in the elderly by enforced bed rest and hospitalization. About a week or 10 days after catheter insertion, formal training with approximately 6 × 1 L bags daily can commence, increasing the fill to 1.5 or 2 L two weeks after insertion. With this unhurried approach to CAPD, leakage is unusual, occurring in only 10% of patients (personal data, unpublished).

In patients presenting as emergencies in ESRD, small volume intermittent peritoneal dialysis (IPD) will permit adequate dialysis, but only if performed for over 12 hours in each 24. As this may involve an overlong stay in bed, a few haemodialyses via a subclavian catheter should be considered, especially in elderly patients, to permit more rapid ambulation and rehabilitation and to avoid venous thromboses. Moreover, many elderly patients can be confused by the two forms of PD – IPD and CAPD – and this may impair their learning process with CAPD. Thus, in general, a brief period of post-insertion catheter flushing (until fluid is no longer blood-stained) is best followed by a break from all forms of PD, irrespective of the clinical state of the elderly patient at catheter insertion.

Even more than in younger patients, CAPD training of the elderly must be tailored to the individual. Ideally this training will have commenced with pre-dialysis counselling including home visits to established patients, visits to the dialysis unit, meetings with nursing staff, and educational material such as books and video films. Such pre-dialysis help is not possible for the patient who presents acutely with ESRD. In that situation tuition is best undertaken between catheter insertion and formal CAPD training 7–10 days later.

Coexisting visual and hearing handicaps often hamper aspects of training such as blood pressure and weight measurement no less than the bag exchange themselves, but can usually be overcome with the aid of electronic sphygmomanometers and scales. Training in CAPD for the visually handicapped has been well described, and the same devices are often useful in the elderly.

Perhaps one of the most difficult aspects of CAPD training in the elderly is the philosophy of personal responsibility for treatment. The young will usually wish to share in medical decision-making, but older patients may be more content to 'let the doctor decide' rather than realize their own individual role in personal well-being.

Complications

Leakage

With the introductory regime for catheter insertion outlined above, early dialysate leakage is not common, but is more frequent in older patients whose wounds heal more slowly. Hence the need for avoiding large volume fills until at least two weeks after catheter insertion. When leakage occurs late, the catheter is doomed and should be removed. Some elderly patients have remarkably little fibrous tissue ingrowth into Dacron cuffs even at 12 months, so firm fixing of the catheter to the skin is essential for many months after insertion.

Peritonitis

'Surgical' peritonitis (perforated viscus, diverticulitis, cholecystitis, appendicitis, etc.) is more common in elderly than in young patients[23]. Hence the need for vigilance in the assessment of peritonitis in elderly CAPD patients. This implies a readiness to perform laparotomy early to exclude a surgical cause; the penalty for late surgery is an unacceptably high mortality from surgical peritonitis[23].

Gram-positive (*Staphylococcus albus, S. aureus*) peritonitis is never associated with a surgical cause, though *S. aureus* peritonitis commonly presents with a rigid abdomen and signs of septic shock. Vigorous resuscitation of such patients with intravenous infusions of plasma and intravenous antibiotics is essential as the sequelae of septic shock in the elderly may be profound with unmasking of underlying vascular disease in the form of myocardial and cerebral ischaemia.

Peritonitis due to Gram-negative organisms should always raise the possibility of a surgical cause. Anaerobes in the PD fluid indicate the need for urgent laparotomy. Diverticulitis can be a difficult diagnostic problem. *E. coli* will be found on culture, but the attack may settle with continued lavage and antibiotics; suspicion of diverticulitis as a cause is aroused when *E. coli* peritonitis recurs in an elderly patient. Sigmoidoscopy and barium enema should be performed; if diverticular disease is confirmed and *E. coli* peritonitis has been frequent, PD should be discontinued and the patient switched to haemodialysis. Peritonitis is no more common overall in the elderly than in the young[24-26].

Hernias

Inguinal, para-umbilical, incisional and epigastric hernias are particularly common in the elderly. They are always exacerbated by CAPD, and should be repaired before starting CAPD. A period of 2–3 months on haemodialysis will allow sound wound healing. Hernias commonly present *de novo* during CAPD, and may initially masquerade as genital swelling[27]. Again, surgical repair and a break from CAPD are generally indicated, although trusses will sometimes prove useful.

Backache

This is common in elderly patients where the inevitable lordotic posture imposed by a full abdomen is inflicted upon an osteoporotic or arthritic spine[28]. If symptoms are intractable, a change from CAPD may be unavoidable.

Underdialysis

Peritoneal mass transport is partly dependent on splanchnic blood flow and is thus reduced in efficiency in the presence of vascular disease[29]. This is a theoretical disadvantage in the elderly but it is surprising how infrequently it poses a problem in practice. In the author's personal experience of CAPD in the elderly, widespread atheroma has only once been associated with underdialysis, while most patients with manifest cardiovascular disease can be successfully treated by CAPD. Early reports of oral dipyridamole enhancing peritoneal clearance of urea and creatinine are intriguing[30,31], but unconfirmed. Alternate methods of improving peritoneal transport mechanisms pharmacologically would be welcome, especially for the elderly.

Loss of ultrafiltration

This problem is no more common in the elderly than in other patients. Its cause is still unknown. Continuing CAPD without dialysate in the peritoneal cavity overnight usually leads to restoration of the ultrafiltration capacity of the peritoneal membrane.

Peripheral vascular disease

Many elderly patients with pre-existing peripheral vascular disease will experience symptoms of reduced distal blood flow when they start CAPD. It has been suggested that this is due to compression of the major blood vessels by the presence of fluid in the abdominal cavity. Rather than being regarded as a contraindication to CAPD this complication should lead to reconstructive surgery whenever possible[28].

Obesity

Although the early weight gain of many malnourished patients treated with CAPD is beneficial, some patients, often elderly women, gain weight progressively and excessively during CAPD and so become obese. The excessive use of hypertonic solution exchanges is a major contributory factor to this problem in those who cannot control their fluid intake; 80–320 g of carbohydrate are typically absorbed from the dialysate each day[32].

Hyperlipidaemia

Hypertriglyceridaemia with elevated very low density lipoproteins is the typical lipid abnormality of uraemia[33]. This abnormality is aggravated by the continuous glucose absorption from peritoneal dialysate. While this may be a theoretical risk factor for the development of atheroma in younger patients, it is highly unlikely to affect significantly the natural history of established vascular disease in the older patient. Hyperlipidaemia is thus best ignored in older patients on CAPD.

Catheter migration

Displacement of the catheter from the pelvis usually presents as poor outflow ('one way obstruction'). The problem is less often seen in older patients because of the less active omentum, but when it does occur it is commonly associated with faecal loading and consequent filling of the pelvis with distended sigmoid loops. In such patients vigorous purging may result in the catheter resuming a normal position but replacement may be necessary. Although the use of catheters other than the straight or curled Tenckhoff catheter may be associated with less migration, personal experience with over 150 standard catheters (in all age groups) indicates that the one third migration rate and 28% failure rate reported by the Toronto group using Tenckhoff catheters is very high, and a malposition rate of 5–10% more typical (personal data, unpublished).

Psychological problems

Few studies have addressed psychological aspects of CAPD in any age group, but it has been suggested that acceptance of changed body image, adjustment to the daily ritual of bag changing and satisfaction with reduced physical capacities are necessary for long-term well-being[17]. In comparison with younger patients, the elderly have a positive advantage with regard to these aspects. Body image, in particular the permanent catheter and bag along with a distended abdomen, has a potential impact on sexuality, and leads many younger patients to dislike CAPD even though renal failure itself impairs libido and sexual performance irrespective of the type of dialysis treatment[34]. However, patients in their seventh and eighth decades of life are usually less concerned than younger patients with sexuality, so the changed body image caused by CAPD rarely poses psychological problems for the elderly.

For most patients, CAPD involves nearly 1500 bag exchanges per year, consuming 500–1000 hours annually on treatment. The day-in, day-out routine is psychologically taxing, and failure to cope with its demands may lead to mistakes in technique causing peritonitis. The elderly are again at an advantage here. Pressures of work and family

84

life will not be present, and the adoption of a less demanding life-style after retirement usually allows the elderly to accommodate the ritual of daily bag changing without major disruption of previous activities.

Elderly patients with ESRD undoubtedly have reduced physical performance, exercise tolerance and general fitness than their peers without renal failure[35,36] but, in common with many other chronic disabling diseases, patients' perception of enjoyment of life does not relate to 'objective' measures of well-being[37]. It has been noted that elderly people with chronic illnesses perceive their own health as superior to others[38], and this 'self-deceptive' perception has positive psychological benefits for the elderly CAPD patient. Others might regard them as merely existing with a greatly reduced life-style, but the patients would see themselves as enjoying life rather than resenting life-prolonging therapy.

Vascular access

Technique failures, largely due to peritonitis, lead to an annual transfer from CAPD to haemodialysis of 10–20% of patients[39-43]. In addition, many patients need shorter periods of haemodialysis during interruption of CAPD when the catheter fails through intractable infection, displacement or leakage. Although short to medium term (1–8 weeks) vascular access for haemodialysis can be obtained easily with a subclavian catheter, a previously constructed arteriovenous fistula proves a major advantage for such patients. As potential treatment failures cannot reliably be identified in advance, it is, in my opinion, wisest to attempt fistula construction in all CAPD patients.

The elderly patient is perhaps a little different owing to the higher prevalence of heart disease. However, as the frequency with which heart failure is acutely exacerbated by a fistula is low, this risk need not preclude fistula construction save in a frail minority. Nonetheless, a fistula will impose increased cardiac workload[44], and regular review of cardiac size and function is essential in such patients. Occasionally a fistula may need to be closed but usually only when CAPD has been reliably established.

RESULTS

Survival

Meaningful survival data of elderly patients on CAPD are scanty. Individual centres have reported relatively short-term results on relatively small groups of patients. Further attempts have been made to compare results with haemodialysis but the whole area of such analyses is bedevilled by the problem of selection of patients. As was mentioned previously, age-specific acceptance rates in patients aged over 65 vary from virtually zero to nearly 100 patients per million population, so that interpretation of survival data can only be meaningful if the acceptance rates for treatment are quoted together with survival data. For example, if centre A accepts 100 patients per million population per year aged over 65, and has a 60% survival at two years, the overall impact on deaths from renal failure in the population is superior to centre B with an acceptance rate of only 50 per million population per year but with an apparently better survival rate of 80% at two years. This is because 60 patients per million population survive two years in community A but only 40 in B. Nonetheless some crude conclusions can be drawn. Nissenson et al.[5] from Los Angeles, California (where one may assume that the age-specific acceptance rate is high) report a survival at two years of around 65% in patients aged over 60 years at the commencement of CAPD – although only 24 of an original cohort of 171 patients were available for analysis. An identical survival rate of 65% at two years was reported by Wu et al. from Toronto[45]. Similar results emerge from the National Institutes of Health CAPD Registry Report (1984) where of over 2000 patients aged over 60 years at the start of CAPD, survival was 70% at 18 months[46]. A recent analysis of results from Newcastle, a pioneer of CAPD, showed a 70% survival at two years in patients aged over 50 years[47]. These figures resemble the author's own early experience with CAPD in the elderly, albeit on a small group of patients[9]. Other published reports on the overall survival of patients on CAPD do not permit calculation of survival of elderly patients.

Rehabilitation and quality of life

In view of the enormous resources involved in ESRD treatment it is both surprising and an indictment of many nephrologists that so little has been published on rehabilitation and quality of life[35,36]. This is particularly so in the case of the elderly patient with renal failure in whom the sceptic might argue that technology is merely providing a postponement of death by a few years at great financial cost and continuing distress to the patient. Fortunately, such uninformed cynicism does not reflect the experience of most nephrologists who, although they may not have collected firm data on quality of life and rehabilitation, are nonetheless convinced that their patients are benefitting from treatment. Furthermore, their patients agree.

Early experience in Sheffield indicated that the majority of patients over 60 years old on CAPD were leading independent lives with no reduction in their activities of daily living compared with their lifestyle before starting dialysis[9]. A comparison of quality of life of patients on CAPD and haemodialysis has been made but this study was restricted to patients under 55 years old[48]. Preliminary data, however, suggested a slightly higher degree of rehabilitation on CAPD. Other studies of quality of life have tried to compare CAPD with other treatments[49] or have analysed the results with respect to case-mix such as race, age, sex and underlying disease[36]. Hardly surprisingly, it has been shown that quality of life is better in younger than older patients[36].

Drop-outs to haemodialysis

For many this is the central ground of debate when results of CAPD are considered. Certainly it is a key area for countries such as the UK where CAPD for the elderly has grown rapidly, as no alternative treatment is available and the long-term planning of hospital haemodialysis for patients no longer able to undertake CAPD is critical[50]. If on the other hand CAPD and haemodialysis in the elderly are seen as complementary rather than competing treatments, a switch of treatment from CAPD to haemodialysis need not be regarded as a bad thing: the term 'treatment failure' has perhaps blinkered rational thought about this aspect of CAPD results. It is manifestly clear, however, that irrespective of age, few patients have remained on CAPD as a sole mode of treatment for very many years[51]. Technique survival in two British units is only 40% at three years taking into account 'drop-outs' by death, transplantation or transfer to haemodialysis[46,50]. Even in the most enthusiastic and experienced units a technique survival rate of above 60% at three years is unlikely[45], and, perhaps surprisingly, the old fare as well as the young[26,43]. Nowhere are there data to suggest that treatment failures are more common in the elderly than in the young; indeed the reverse may be the case although this is not yet established[52].

Hospitalization

Over 50% of patients on CAPD need hospitalization within their first year on treatment[24] and 70% by 18 months[46]. There is no difference between patients younger and older than 60 years nor indeed between diabetics and non-diabetics[24,46,53]. The majority of hospital admissions are due to episodes of peritonitis or catheter-related problems, although in the elderly there is an additional burden of hospitalization for other conditions such as gastrointestinal or cardiac diseases[26]. As a result, older patients spend longer in hospital than do younger patients on CAPD (personal data, unpublished) and in patients aged over 60 years on CAPD an average of 10–14 days in hospital per year is to be expected, even if treatment for peritonitis is given at home after the initial period of hospital assessment[46].

COMPARISONS WITH HAEMODIALYSIS

This area is fraught with difficulty. No prospective, randomized, controlled trials comparing CAPD and haemodialysis have been published nor are they ever likely as such trials would be impossible to conduct or interpret. A retrospective analysis of data from the Registry of the European Dialysis and Transplant Association has been performed to compare CAPD and haemodialysis examining paired patients from the database matched for age, sex, primary renal disease, body weight and age at onset of renal replacement therapy[54]. Unfortunately, this analysis could not take into account the characteristics which might have governed the initial clinical choice of CAPD or haemodialysis clinical therapy for an individual patient. The data suggested, however, an inferior survival of patients on CAPD compared with haemodialysis and matched for sex, age, primary renal disease and country of origin. Similar conclusions were drawn in Mion's unit where, despite their great experience of PD, results obtained with CAPD were inferior to those with haemodialysis[55]. Nonetheless, within a single renal unit, analysis by the Cox proportional hazard method to adjust for selection bias suggested that CAPD and haemodialysis offer similar life expectancy[56]. In other studies too, similar survival and rehabilitation have been found in CAPD and haemodialysis patients[49,57,58].

Hospitalization seems to be more common in CAPD patients than in haemodialysis patients[53]. In view of the enhanced risk of hospitalization in the elderly mentioned above, the highest rate of hospitalization is to be expected in elderly CAPD patients. It has been suggested that rehabilitation and quality of life of CAPD patients is inferior to that of haemodialysis patients[36] but no paper has specifically addressed the question of quality of life in elderly CAPD patients compared with elderly haemodialysis patients. One must bear in mind the excellent results obtained with haemodialysis in the elderly in the USA and Europe[18,59–61], where a 5-year survival of 40–50% in the over-60s is typical. In terms of survival, rehabilitation, physical performance and perceived health, the results are outstanding and ought to serve as a yardstick for future comparisons of results of CAPD in the elderly. Indeed, some units regard haemodialysis as safer and preferable to CAPD in the elderly[4], despite the tide of opinion currently favouring CAPD.

ALTERNATIVE PERITONEAL DIALYSIS STRATEGIES

Several alternative peritoneal dialysis strategies are available. Some elderly patients are unsuitable for CAPD, because of inability to cope with the repetitive tedium of bag changing, and for haemodialysis through lack of vascular access. In such patients alternative peritoneal

89

dialysis strategies can be considered. Although largely discarded as a chronic treatment, intermittent peritoneal dialysis can prove useful for those patients with residual renal function (GFR > 1–2 ml/min). Below that level of residual renal function results are likely to be poor, attended by underdialysis and malnutrition[62] and this is likely to prove rapidly fatal in the elderly patient. Continuous cyclic peritoneal dialysis (CCPD) has not yet been widely applied to elderly patients. However, in view of the need for a regular routine and attachment to a cycler every night it is perhaps a form of treatment more suited to the elderly patient than the younger patient and by avoiding the tedium of daily bag exchanges may prove a sensible option for a selected group of patients[63]. Long-term results in different categories of patients are eagerly awaited.

RESOURCES NEEDED FOR A CAPD PROGRAMME IN THE ELDERLY

In view of the large number of patients who switch to haemodialysis from CAPD it is unreasonable to attempt CAPD in the elderly without free access to a hospital dialysis programme. Initial experience with CAPD in the elderly suggested that, in the short term, hospital haemodialysis facilities would not be greatly stretched by these CAPD 'drop-outs'[9], but more recent experience indicates that in the longer term the demand for hospital haemodialysis will grow despite the widespread use of CAPD[50].

How great is this impact likely to be for countries like the UK and much of Eastern Europe, which have severely limited hospital haemodialysis facilities and which tend to exclude the elderly from renal replacement programmes[12]? Approximately 20 patients aged over 60 years per million total population per year are accepted onto dialysis in Sweden, Belgium and Switzerland[59], and 20/million population/year is roughly the difference in flow of new patients which separates European countries with high and low acceptance rates for dialysis[64]. If one assumes that all these over-60s are initially treated by CAPD; that the long-term technique survival of CAPD is 50%, with 25% drop-out in year 1, 15% in year 2, 10% in year 3, 5% in year 4, then negligible (optimistic figures); that only 50% of transfers to haemodialysis can be treated at home (very optimistic); that few elderly patients are transplanted; that catheter life averages 18 months, with three weeks of haemodialysis treatment before a new catheter is inserted; and that the annual death rate for those aged over 60 years is 15% – with all these reasonable assumptions, based on available data, how many hospital haemodialysis sessions will be needed per million population?

Figure 4.3 shows that the steady state CAPD pool would be 80 with 12 deaths per year (15%), 8 patients would go onto haemodialysis

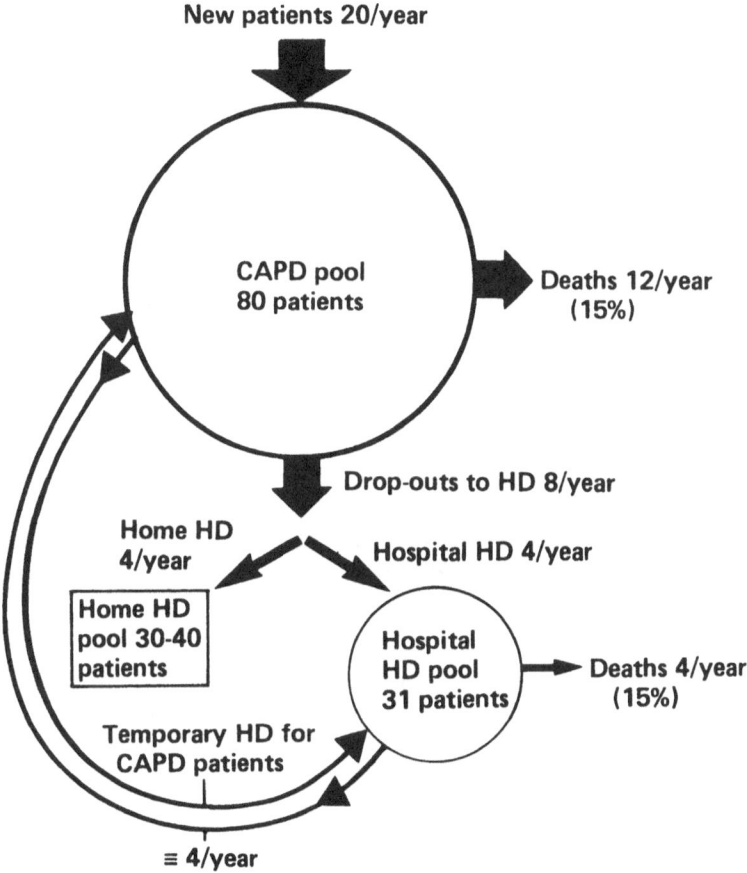

FIGURE 4.3 Steady-state model of haemodialysis (HD) requirements necessary for a CAPD programme for patients aged over 60 years of age (see text for details). Numbers relate to a population base of one million total population (all ages)

annually, 4 to home haemodialysis and 4 to hospital haemodialysis. If the death rate on hospital haemodialysis remained 15% per annum, in the steady state there would be 27 patients over the age of 60 per million population on hospital haemodialysis, with an additional haemodialysis work-load of over 200 patient-weeks annually to provide temporary haemodialysis between changes of catheter. This makes a total of 31 hospital haemodialysis spaces per million population for those aged over 60 years, equivalent to five or eight dialysis stations depending on whether four or six shifts use each station per week. In the UK this is not far short of the *total* hospital haemodialysis capacity of most units. Without a CAPD programme the need would be more than double, nearly 70 spaces per million population even if 50% of the 20 new patients annually were capable of home haemodialysis.

CONCLUSIONS

This review has attempted to analyse current results of CAPD therapy in elderly patients and certain broad conclusions can be drawn. Where no haemodialysis facilities for the elderly exist, CAPD is for most patients preferable to death, and for many patients a superior form of treatment to haemodialysis. There is little evidence yet that there are major differences in outcome for large groups of elderly patients on either form of treatment, as judged by survival, rehabilitation, or quality of life (subjectively or objectively assessed). However, the best published reports of haemodialysis in the elderly are outstandingly good and are as yet not matched by CAPD.

Costs have not been discussed in detail but deserve a mention. CAPD is roughly equivalent in cost to home haemodialysis and both are considerably cheaper than hospital haemodialysis[65]. However, many elderly patients cannot be treated by home haemodialysis, so in cost-effective terms it is reasonable to offer CAPD before hospital haemodialysis to most elderly patients provided inability to cope with CAPD, frequent peritonitis, dissatisfaction with treatment, poor dialysis and other technique failures are recognized early and hospital haemodialysis then provided. With such an integrated approach, those who remain on CAPD should do well, and the increased costs for those on hospital haemodialysis can be justified by the good outcome that should be attainable for them. Attempts to define the 'gold standard' of renal replacement therapy are likely to prove futile for the elderly, as no one form of treatment could be expected to be universally acceptable; CAPD and haemodialysis are complementary, rather than rival, treatments.

The widespread use of CAPD in the elderly has come at a time when the philosophy behind renal replacement therapy has radically changed. In the 1970s, dialysis evolved as a treatment for young fit patients awaiting transplantation and even on dialysis good rehabilitation was achieved. Since then, as Quevedo et al.[66] have recently pointed out, 'older, sicker and often indigent patients were dialysed; fatal uremia was converted to a chronic illness', and they continue 'powerful, costly technology delays death, but results in chronic illnesses that we barely understand'. Nonetheless, despite an apparent poor quality of life, elderly patients on dialysis share with other patient groups a psychosocial adaptation to illness which preserves their own perceived quality of life[37].

Any discussion of CAPD in the elderly would be incomplete without considering the issue of withdrawal of treatment. It has been reported that as many as 1 in 6 of patients aged over 60 years die from discontinuing dialysis[67,68]. This usually occurs after irreversible nonfatal brain damage, mostly due to cerebrovascular disease, but in a significant minority of patients no medical or psychiatric cause for stopping dialysis is evident[67]. Presumably such patients are tired of life, their treatment or both. Withdrawal of dialysis imposes stress and guilt feelings on both family members and dialysis staff[68], but must be viewed dispassionately as a real option for elderly patients on both CAPD and haemodialysis.

Renal replacement therapy ought to be offered to all who can benefit from it, irrespective of age; currently, for many elderly patients CAPD is the only option open to them. Such patients need not fear such a Hobson's choice, for in only 10 years CAPD already rivals haemodialysis for both young and old alike.

ACKNOWLEDGEMENTS

Grateful thanks are due to Ms Virginia Newton, Medical Librarian, Royal Devon and Exeter Hospital.

93

REFERENCES

1. Gurland, H. J., Brunner, F. B., Chantler, C., Donckerwolcke, R. A., Jacobs, C., Kramer, P. and Wing, A. J. (1976). Combined report on regular dialysis and transplantation in Europe VI, 1975. *Proc. Eur. Dial. Transplant Assoc.*, **13**, 3–58
2. Mion, C. M., Mourad, B., Canaud, B., Chong, G., Polito, C., Oules, R., Branger, B., Granolleras, C., Issautier, R., Slingeneyer, A., Ramperez, P., Flavier, J-L., Deschodt, G., Emond, C., Cosette, P., Florence, P., Chouzenoux, R., Huchard, G., Fitte, H., Marty, L., Grolleau-Raoux, R. and Shaldon, S. (1983). Maintenance dialysis: a survey of 17 years' experience in Languedoc–Roussillon with a comparison of methods in 'standard population'. *Am. Soc. Artif. Intern. Organs J.*, **6**, 205–13
3. Shapiro, F. L. and Umen, A. J. (1983). Risk factors in hemodialysis patient survival. *Am. Soc. Artif. Intern. Organs J.* , **6**, 176–81
4. Annual Report. (1982). Renal Network Coordinating Council of the Upper Midwest. *Endstage Renal Disease Network*, **7**, 80–97
5. Nissenson, A. R., Gentile, D. E., Soderblom, R. E., Oliver, D. F. and Brax, C. (1986). Morbidity and mortality of continuous ambulatory peritoneal dialysis: regional experience and long-term prospects. *Am. J. Kidney Dis.*, **7**, 229–34
6. Popovitch, R. P., Moncrief, J. W., Decherd, J. P., Bomar, B. and Pyle, W. K. (1976). The definition of a novel portable/wearable equilibrium peritoneal dialysis technique. *Abstracts Am. Soc. Artif. Intern. Organs*, **6**, 64
7. Oreopoulos, D. G., Robson, M., Izatt, S., Clayton, S. and deVeber, G. A. (1978). A simple and safe technique for continuous ambulatory peritoneal dialysis (CAPD). *Trans. Am. Soc. Artif. Intern. Organs*, **24**, 484–87
8. Deber, R. B., Blidner, I. N., Carr, L. M. and Barnsley, J. M. (1985). The impact of selected patient characteristics on practitioners' treatment recommendations for end-stage renal disease. *Med. Care*, **23**, 95–109
9. Nicholls, A. J., Waldek, S., Platts, M. M., Moorhead, P. J. and Brown, C. B. (1984). Impact of continuous ambulatory peritoneal dialysis on treatment of renal failure in patient aged over 60. *Br. Med. J.*, **288**, 18–9
10. Friedman, E. A. (1984). Critical appraisal of continuous ambulatory peritoneal dialysis. *Ann. Rev. Med.*, **35**, 233–48
11. Warner, K. E. (1975). A 'desperation–reaction' model of medical diffusion. *Health Serv Res.*, **10**, 369–83
12. Brunner, F. P., Broyer, M., Brynger, H., Challah, S., Fassbinder, W., Oules, R., Rizzoni, G., Selwood, N. H. and Wing, A. J. (1985). Combined report on regular dialysis and transplantation in Europe, XV, (1984). *Proc. Eur. Dial. Transplant Assoc. – ERA*, **22**, 5–53
13. Broyer, M., Brunner, F. P., Brynger, H., Fassbinder, W., Guillou, P. J., Oules, R., Rizzoni, G., Selwood, N. H., Wing, A. J., Challah, S. and Dykes, S. R. (1986). Demography of dialysis and transplantation in Europe, 1984. *Nephrol. Dial. Transplant.*, **1**, 1–8
14. Mion, C., Slingeneyer, A., Canaud, B., Mourad, G., Chong, G., Beraud, J. J., Oules, R. and Branger, B. (1985). The benefits and proper role of CAPD. *Contrib. Nephrol.*, **44**, 148–62
15. Rubin, L. J. and Gutman, R. A. (1978). Hypotension during haemodialysis. *Kidney*, **11**, 21–4

16. Flynn, C. T. and Shadur, C. A. (1981). A comparison of CAPD in diabetics and nondiabetics. *Am. J. Kidney Dis.*, **1**, 15–23
17. Gonsalves–Ebrahim, L., Gulledge, A. D. and Miga, S. (1982). Continuous ambulatory peritoneal dialysis: psychological factors. *Psychosomatics*, **23**, 944–9
18. Westlie, L., Umen, S., Nestrud, S. and Kjellstrand, C. M. (1984). Mortality, morbidity, and life satisfaction in the very old dialysis patient. *Trans. Am. Soc. Artif. Intern. Organs*, **30**, 21–9
19. Shaldon, S., Koch, K. M., Quellhorst, E., Lonnemann, G. and Dinarello, C. A. (1985). CAPD is a second-class treatment. *Contrib. Nephrol.*, **44**, 163–72
20. Ash, S. R., Wolf, G. C. and Bloch, R. (1981). Placement of the Tenckhoff peritoneal dialysis catheter under peritoneoscopic visualisation. *Dial. Transplant.*, **5**, 383–86
21. Ash, S. R., Slingeneyer, A. and Schardin, K. E. (1983). Peritoneal access using the column-disc catheter. *Perspect. Perit. Dial.*, **1**, 9–11
22. Oreopoulos, D. G., Zellerman, G. and Izatt, S. (1979). The Toronto Western Hospital permanent peritoneal catheter and continuous ambulatory peritoneal dialysis connector. In Legrain, M. (ed) *Continuous Ambulatory Peritoneal Dialysis*, pp. 73–81. (New York: Elsevier)
23. Rottembourg, J., Gahl, G. M., Poignet, J. L., Mertani, E., Strippoli, P., Langlois, P., Tranbaloc, P. and Legrain, M. (1983). Severe abdominal complications in patients undergoing continuous ambulatory peritoneal dialysis. *Proc. Eur. Dial. Transplant Assoc.*, **20**, 236–41
24. Wing, A. J., Broyer, M., Brunner, F. P., Brynger, H., Challah, S., Donckerwolcke, R. A., Gretz, N., Jacobs, C., Kramer, P. and Selwood, N. H. (1983). Combined report on regular dialysis and transplantation in Europe, XII, (1982). *Proc. Eur. Dial. Transplant Assoc.*, **20**, 5–71
25. Fragola, J. A., Grube, S., Von Bloch, L. and Bourke, E. (1983). Multicentre study of physical activity and employment status of continuous ambulatory peritoneal dialysis (CAPD) patients in the United States. *Proc. Eur. Dial. Transplant Assoc.*, **20**, 243–9
26. Rubin, J., Kirchner, K., Ray, R. and Bower, J. D. (1985). Demographic factors associated with dialysis technique failures among patients undergoing continuous ambulatory peritoneal dialysis. *Arch. Intern. Med.*, **145**, 1041–4
27. Cooper, J. C., Nicholls, A. J., Simms, J. M., Platts, M. M., Brown, C. B. and Johnson, A. G. (1983). Genital oedema in patients treated by continuous ambulatory peritoneal dialysis: an unusual presentation of inguinal hernia. *Br. Med. J.*, **286**, 1923–4
28. Oreopoulos, D. G. and Khanna, R. (1981). Complications of peritoneal dialysis other than peritonitis. In Nolph K. D. (ed) *Peritoneal Dialysis*, pp. 309–43. (London:Martinus Nijhoff)
29. Nolph, K. D., Stoltz, M. L. and Maher, J. F. (1973). Altered peritoneal permeability in patients with systemic vasculitis. *Ann. Intern. Med.*, **75**, 753–5
30. Ryckelynck, J. P., Pierre, D., DeMartin, A. and Rottembourg, J. (1978). Ameliortion des clairances peritoneales par le dipyridamole. *Nouv. Presse Med.*, **7**, 742
31. Maher, J. F., Hirszel, P., Abraham, J. E., Galen, M. A., Chamberlain, M. and Hohnadel, D. C. (1977). The effect of dipyridamole on peritoneal mass transport. *Trans. Am. Soc. Artif. Intern. Organs*, **23**, 219–24
32. De Santon, N. G., Capodicasa, G., Senatore, R., Cichetti, T., Cirillo, D.,

Damiano, M., Torella, R., Gughiano, D., Improta, L. and Giordano, C. (1979). Glucose utilisation from dialysate in patients on continuous ambulatory peritoneal dialysis. *Intern. J. Artif. Organs*, **2**, 119–24

33. Nicholls, A. J., Cumming, A. M., Catto, G. R. D., Edward, N. and Engeset, J. (1981). Lipid relationships in dialysis and renal transplant patient. *Q. J. Med.*, **50**, 149–60
34. Kanis, J. A. and Nicholls, A. J. (1984). Endocrinology and renal disease. In Keynes, W. M., Fowler, P. B. S. (eds) *Clinical Endocrinology*, pp. 370–408. (London:Heinemann)
35. Johnson, J. P., McCanley, C. R. and Copley, J. B. (1982). The quality of life of hemodialysis and transplant patients. *Kidney Int.*, **22**, 286–91
36. Evans, R. W., Manninen, D. L., Carrison, L. P. Jnr, Hart, L. G., Blagg, C. R., Guman, R. A., Hull, A. R. and Lowrie, E. G. (1985). The quality of life of patients with end-stage renal disease. *N. Engl. J. Med.*, **312**, 553–9
37. Cassileth, B. R., Lusk, E. J., Strouse, T. B., Miller, D. S., Brown, L. L., Cross, P. A. and Tenaglia, A. N. (1984). Psychosocial status in chronic illness: a comparative analysis of six diagnostic groups. *N. Engl. J. Med.*, **311**, 506–11
38. Cockerham, W. C., Sharp, K. and Wilcox, J. A. (1983). Aging and perceived health status. *J. Gerontol.*, **38**, 349–55
39. Oreopoulos, D. G., Khanna, R., Williams, P. and Vas, S. I. (1982). Continuous ambulatory peritoneal dialysis – 1981. *Nephron*, **30**, 293–303
40. Nolph, K. D., Boen, F. S. T., Farrel, P. C. and Pyle, K. W. (1983). Continuous ambulatory peritoneal dialysis in Australia, Europe and the United States: 1981. *Kidney Int.*, **23**, 3–8
41. Prowant, B., Nolph, K. D., Dutton, S., Van Stone, J., Whittier, Fe., Ross, G. Jr. and Moore, H. (1983). Actuarial analysis of patient survival and dropout with various end-stage renal disease therapies. *Am. J. Kidney Dis.*, **3**, 27–31
42. Ramos, J. M., Gokal, R., Siamopolous, K., Ward, M. K., Wilkinson, R. and Kerr, D. N. S. (1983). Continuous ambulatory peritoneal dialysis: three years' experience. *Q. J. Med.*, **206**, 165–86
43. Nolph, K. D., Cutler, S. J., Steinberg, S. M. and Novak, J. W. (1985). Continuous ambulatory peritoneal dialysis in the United States. A three year study. *Kidney Int.*, **28**, 198–205
44. Von Bibra, H., Castro, L., Autenrieth, G., McLeod, A. and Gurland, H. J. (1978). The effects of arteriovenous shunts on cardiac function in dialysis patients – an echocardiographic evaluation. *Clin. Nephrol.*, **9**, 205–9
45. Wu, G., Khanna, R., Vas, S. I., Digenis, G. and Oreopoulos, D. G. (1984). Continuous ambulatory peritoneal dialysis: no longer experimental. *Can. Med. Assoc. J.*, **130**, 699–707
46. Steinberg, S. M., Cutler, S. J., Nolph, K. D. and Novak, J. W. (1984). A comprehensive report on the experience of patients on continuous ambulatory peritoneal dialysis for the treatment of end-stage renal disease. *Am. J. Kidney Dis.*, **4**, 233–41
47. Heaton, A., Rodger, R. S. C., Sellars, L., Goodship, T. H. J., Fletcher, K., Nikolakakis, N., Ward, M. K., Wilkinson, R. and Kerr, D. N. S. (1986). Continuous ambulatory peritoneal dialysis after the honeymoon: review of experience in Newcastle 1979–84. *Br. Med. J.*, **293**, 938–41
48. Simmons, R. G., Anderson, C. and Kamstra, L. (1984). Comparison of quality of life of patients on continuous ambulatory peritoneal dialysis, hemodialysis and transplantation. *Am. J. Kidney Dis.*, **3**, 253–5

49. Charytan, C., Spinowitz, B. S. and Galler, M. (1986). A comparative study of continuous ambulatory peritoneal dialysis and center hemodialysis. Efficacy, complications, and outcome in the treatment of end-stage renal disease. *Arch. Intern. Med.*, **146**, 1138–43

50. Morgan, A. G. and Burden, R. P. (1986). Effect of continuous peritoneal dialysis on a British renal unit. *Br. Med. J.*, **293**, 935–7

51. Coles, G. A. Is peritoneal dialysis a good long-term treatment? *Br. Med. J.*, **290**, 1164–6

52. Oreopoulos, D. G. (1987). Continuous ambulatory peritoneal dialysis. *Br. Med. J.*, **294**, 54

53. Carlson, D. M., Duncan, D. A., Naessens, J. M. and Johnson, W. J. (1984). Hospitalisation in dialysis patients. *Mayo Clin. Proc.*, **59**, 769–75

54. Kramer, P., Broyer, M., Brunner, F. P., Brynger, H., Challah, S., Oules, R., Rozzoni, G., Selwood, N. H., Wing, A. J. and Balas, E. A. (1984). Combined report on regular dialysis and transplantation in Europe, XIV, 1983. *Proc. Eur. Dial. Transplant Assoc. – ERA*, **21**, 5–63

55. Mion, C., Oules, R., Canaud, B., Mourad, G., Slingeneyer, A., Branger, B., Granolleras, C., Al Sabadani, B., Florence, P., Chouzenoux, R., Maurice, F., Issantier, R., Flavier, F. L., Polito, C., Saunier, F., Marty, L., Fontainer, P., Emond, C., Ramtoolah, H., de Cornelissen, F., Huchard, G., Fitte, H. and Boudet, R. (1984). Maintenance dialysis in the elderly. A review of 15 years' experience in Languedoc–Roussillon. *Proc. Eur. Dial. Transplant Assoc. – ERA*, **21**, 490–509

56. Burton, P. R. and Walls, J. (1986). Population-adjusted survival on haemodialysis and continuous ambulatory peritoneal dialysis. *Nephrol. Dial. Tranplant.*, **1**, 111 (Abstr.)

57. Gokal, R., Baillod, R., Bogle, S., Hunt, L., Jakubowski, C., Marsh, F., Ogg, C., Oliver, D., Ward, M. and Wilkinson, R. (1987). Multicentre study on outcome of treatment in patients on CAPD and haemodialysis. *Nephrol. Dial. Transplant.*, **2**, 172–178

58. Capelli, J. P., Canniscioli, T. C., Vallorani, R. D. and Bobeck, J. D. (1985). Comparative analysis of survival on home hemodialysis, in-center hemodialysis and chronic peritoneal dialysis, and chronic peritoneal dialysis (CAPD-IPD) therapies. *Dial. Transplant.*, **14**, 38–58

59. Jacobs, C., Diallo, A., Balas, E. A., Nectoux, M. and Etienne, S. (1984). Maintenance haemodialysis treatment in patients aged over 60 years. Demographic profile, clinical aspects and outcome. *Proc. Eur. Dial. Transplant Assoc.*, **21**, 477–489

60. Schaefer, K., Asmus, G., Quellhorst, E., Pauls, A., Von Herrath, D. and Jahnke, J. (1984). Optimum dialysis treatment for patients over 60 years with primary renal disease. Survival data and clinical results from 242 patients treated either by haemodialysis or haemofiltration. *Proc. Eur. Dial. Transplant Assoc.*, **21**, 510–17

61. Chester, A. C., Rakowski, T. A., Argy, W. P. Jr., Gaicalone, A. and Schreiner, G. E. (1979). Hemodialysis in the eighth and ninth decades of life. *Arch. Intern. Med.*, **139**, 1001–1006

62. Ahmad, S., Shen, F-H. and Blagg, C. R. (1981). Intermittent peritoneal dialysis as renal replacement therapy. In Nolph K. D. ed *Peritoneal Dialysis*, pp. 144–177. (London: Martinus Nijhoff)

63. Diaz-Buxo, J. A., Walker, P. J., Farmer, C. D., Chandler, J. T., Holt, K. L. and Cox, P. (1981). Continuous cyclic peritoneal dialysis. *Trans. Am. Soc. Artif. Intern. Organs*, **27**, 51–4
64. European Dialysis and Transplant Association Registry. Demography of dialysis and transplantation in Europe, 1984. (1986). *Nephrol. Dial. Transplant.*, **1**, 1–8
65. Stason, W. B. and Barnes, B. A. (1985). *The Effectiveness and Costs of Continuous Ambulatory Peritoneal Dialysis* (CAPD), (Health Technology Case Study 35; publication no. OTA-HCS-35). (Washington, D.C: Office of Technology Assessment)
66. Quevedo, S. G., Young, J. H., Carrie, B. J. and Holman, H. R. (1986). Continuous ambulatory peritoneal dialysis: bridging the gap between evaluation and practice in chronic illness. *Ann. Intern. Med.*, **104**, 430–2
67. Neu, S. and Kjellstrand, C. M. (1986). Stopping long-term dialysis. An empirical study of withdrawal of life-supporting treatment. *N. Engl. J. Med.*, **314**, 14–20
68. Rodin, G. M., Chmara, J., Ennis, J., Fenton, S., Locking, H. and Steinhouse, K. (1981). Stopping life-sustaining medical treatment: psychiatric considerations in the termination of renal dialysis. *Can. J. Psychiatry*, **26**, 540–4

5
CAPD IN CHILDREN

R. A. BAILLOD

INTRODUCTION

After successful renal transplantation, CAPD has proved to be the most rewarding treatment available for children with end-stage renal failure (ESRF). Its use in infants has made future transplantation a reality. Haemodialysis has been used successfully in children since the late 1960s[1] but is technically difficult and symptomatically very unpleasant during the treatments, especially in small children with blood volumes under two litres. Very few paediatric dialysis centres existed and fewer had sufficient skills to teach with confidence home haemodialysis or even the less technically difficult treatment of home intermittent peritoneal dialysis, IPD. As a result, patients were either hospitalized for prolonged periods or had to make long journeys for treatment whilst awaiting transplantation. In some instances families moved house in order to obtain treatment. Family life, schooling and work were seriously disrupted as one of the parents usually stayed at the hospital with the child. CAPD is definitely a home-based treatment. The diet, although not free, is more normal than the diet for haemodialysis or IPD, and the dangers of acute fluid overload or lethal potassium levels are rarely encountered. Its simplicity makes it relatively non-intrusive and all members of the family can live a near normal life.

Historical note

IPD, although used to treat children with ESRF since 1967[2], has never been widely used. The EDTA annual report of 1979[3] quotes that only 38, or 4.6%, of 832 children on dialysis in Europe were treated by IPD. CAPD was first devised in 1976[4]. Moncrief and Nolph in their original report on CAPD drew attention to its particular value for children and infants. In 1980 the first abstract on CAPD in children appeared[5]. By 1981 more extensive experience was available and definitive data showed that it was a more suitable dialysis treatment for children. The special value of CAPD for infants was apparent as early as 1981[6,7].

PATIENTS UNSUITABLE FOR CAPD

Having stated firmly the preference for CAPD above all other methods of dialysis in children, there are situations when CAPD cannot be undertaken. The most serious problem is lack of peritoneal cavity as can result from multiple surgery. Pylonephritis with obstructive uropathy and hypoplasia account for almost one third of children requiring renal replacement therapy[8]. These children often require surgery. Provided this surgery is retroperitoneal, the peritoneum remains intact. However, some surgery is transperitoneal and may have been complicated by infections leading to loss of the peritoneal cavity. Adhesions may produce 'pockets' of peritoneum which do not allow adequate drainage. The presence of an anterior abdominal wall ureterostomy or ileal conduit may add to the risk of infections of the peritoneal catheter tunnel and peritonitis during CAPD treatment. A careful history and examination of past notes and operation sheets are necessary to make the correct decision.

Peritonitis is the principal problem with CAPD. Most primary infections of the peritoneum can be traced to a technical error and breakdown of technique, although subsequent infections with the same peritoneal catheter *in situ* may arise without further technical errors. CAPD treatment is technically easy but carelessness may cause disaster. Not only is peritonitis excruciatingly painful, but it can be lethal if not treated urgently. Unfortunately, not all children have caring and responsible parents. Should there be genuine doubt about parents' ability, it is unkind and dangerous to allow such adults to undertake CAPD treatment.

WHEN TO START TREATMENT

Infants

Although some infants present with anuria and acutely deranged biochemistry which clearly needs urgent correction, many more have a degree of renal failure which can be managed by diet, drugs and careful electrolyte balance. They have sufficient urine output to allow adequate fluid balance and feeding. These infants can be treated conservatively for long periods despite very low creatinine clearances but they do not grow[9]. It has been shown that failure to grow after ensuring optimum dietary intake is the most important factor to indicate that dialysis should be started. An infant should grow 36 cm in the first two years of life and the head circumference should increase by 13 cm in the same period. Failure to grow is all the more significant since there is also loss of cerebral growth and mental retardation[10–12]. There can be no harm in inserting a peritoneal catheter early in this group of patients, allowing it to heal for a minimum of three weeks and then electively starting dialysis.

Children

For patients and parents who are warned that renal replacement will eventually be necessary, the aspect of dialysis is always wished away! Children are very tolerant of uraemic state and appear to have minimal or no symptoms. The long-term loss of appetite associated with renal failure makes the transition to ESRF much more insidious; the gradual loss of health is often only appreciated after improvement in health had been brought about by dialysis. The doctor may be the first to lose his nerve as he sees the worsening biochemistry, lack of growth and increasing evidence of hyperparathyroid disease.

It is good practice to place the peritoneal catheter well in advance on two accounts. Firstly, it makes the operation, anaesthetic and post-operative periods safer and secondly, it allows healing of the abdominal wound and sealing of the tunnel. One month prior to dialysis would be ideal.

TECHNICAL ASPECTS

The simplicity of peritoneal dialysis resulted in its historically being relegated to the inexperienced junior medical and nursing staff. Its long-term success, however, is dependent on meticulous technique in the placement of the peritoneal catheter and prevention of infection. It is difficult for staff to recognize that it requires much higher standards of sterile technique than is necessary for haemodialysis. This arises from the fact that when the peritoneum is filled with dialysis fluid it is the perfect culture medium, being maintained at body temperature with all the necessary nutrients of sugar from the dialysis fluid, amino acids and protein from the patient.

The bacterial cultures of peritonitis are predominantly skin organisms demonstrating that the infections enter the peritoneum via the catheter, either down the internal lumen or around the catheter through the tunnel. Infection can be introduced at operation or during the healing period, especially if there is leakage of dialysis fluid through the wound and into the tunnel. It is often impossible to eradicate infection from foreign bodies such as the catheter. Operative techniques and post-operative management must be perfect if immediate and long-term infection are to be avoided. Thereafter, education in the recognition of inadvertent breakdown in technique and how to deal with the problem immediately are the factors vital for success. In the child these comments are of greater significance. Delay in treatment will lead not only to sepsis or loss of the peritoneum but to loss of life if haemodialysis cannot be instituted.

Catheter insertion

Preliminary examination of the abdomen

Development of a hernia or enlargement of an existing hernia can occur when volumes of fluid are left in the abdomen of ambulatory patients[13]. Careful examination must be made of the usual hernial sites in groin or umbilicus, with plans to repair any found at the time of operation. Inspection of previous surgical scars and ureterostomies is necessary to assess if a good technical result can be achieved.

Choice of catheter

The straight two-cuffed Tenckhoff seems to have survived all new designs. The 'circular looped' Tenckhoff catheter is favoured by some units. The Lifecath seems to be particularly unsuitable for the very young as the bowel can be caught and twisted around it, causing obstruction and sepsis[14]. The intra-abdominal section of the peritoneal catheter does not have to be too long or placed deeply in the pelvis to get good drainage as the system is closed syphonage. The shorter the catheter, the less area there is for slime formation and potential infection. Long catheters often lie up against the bladder or rectum, giving discomfort. It is possible to purchase catheters with loose cuffs which can then be glued into selected positions. The glue takes 72 hours to fix. An active dialysis unit can make up a series of catheters with different cuff site positions and then choose a catheter appropriate to each child.

Anaesthetic

The operation must be performed in an operating theatre with a general anaesthetic and intubation. Intubation is necessary as almost all children will need to have inspection and possible removal of a section of their omentum; some handling of the intestines thus inevitably occurs.

103

The omentum

The omentum in children is a fine, mobile structure, which attacks and wraps itself around the catheter (Figures 5.1–5.3). At the operation it should be examined and if large and extending into the pelvis its lower edge should be removed[15].

The incision

The standard longitudinal incision through the linea alba leads to incisional hernia in many children[13,16]. Transverse incisions, which grow with the child, are standard today, especially in very small children. In infants the bladder extends almost up to the umbilicus causing the peritoneum to be folded upon itself. Failure to recognize this or get good closure of the peritoneum leads to dialysate leaks into the pelvic floor and scrotum. For this reason it may be necessary to make the incision level with the umbilicus in small babies.

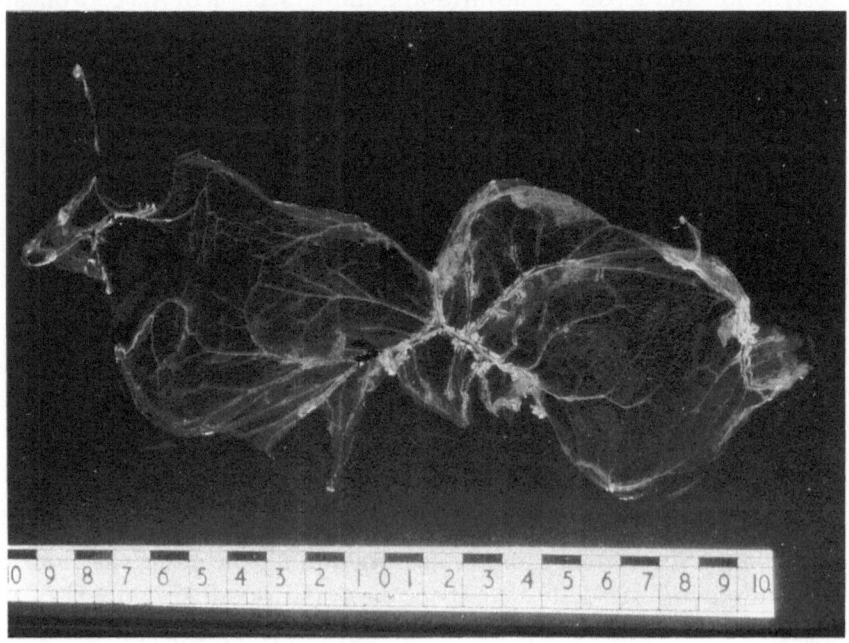

FIGURE 5.1 The omentum of a six-week-old baby

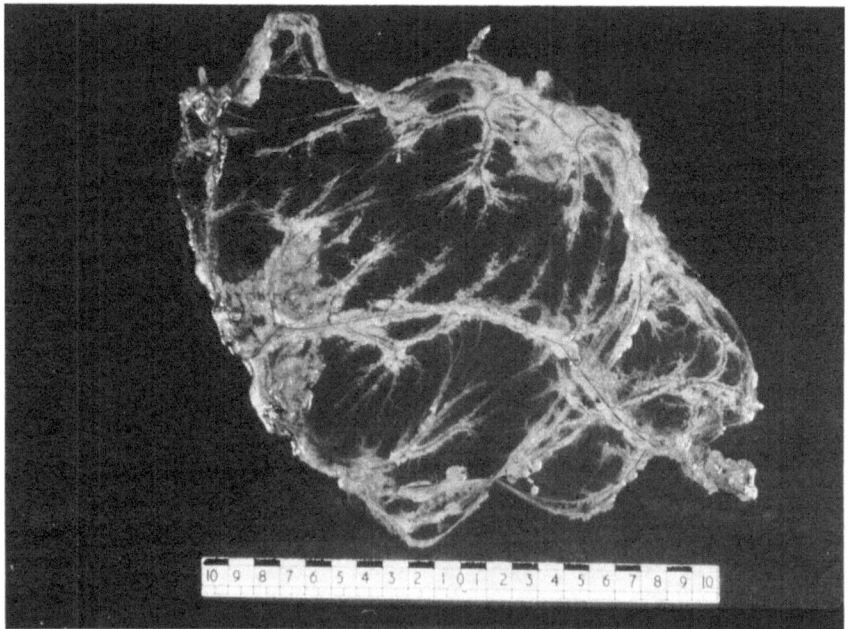

FIGURE 5.2 The omentum of a nine-year-old boy. These fine tissues always wrap themselves around and obstruct the catheters shortly after placement

Operation

The technique used by myself for the past four years is described below. It is based on 18 years of personal experience in placing silastic catheters in 370 patients aged 6 weeks to 81 years old[17].

The peritoneum is approached by an incision along the lateral border of the rectus muscle in the right or left lower quadrant of the abdomen. In infants the approach is via a transverse skin incision, lateral and just below the umbilicus. The edge of the rectus sheath is seen and the anterior sheath is incised along its border. Retraction of the rectus abdominis muscle reveals the posterior rectus sheath and parietal peritoneum beneath. A small opening of 2 cm is made in the peritoneum under the rectus muscle. After inspection of the omentum and its partial removal, a malleable copper spatula is inserted if necessary to protect the peritoneal contents. A spiked introducer is used to pierce the catheter through the intact rectus sheath. The peritoneum stretches to form a neck which can angle the catheter.

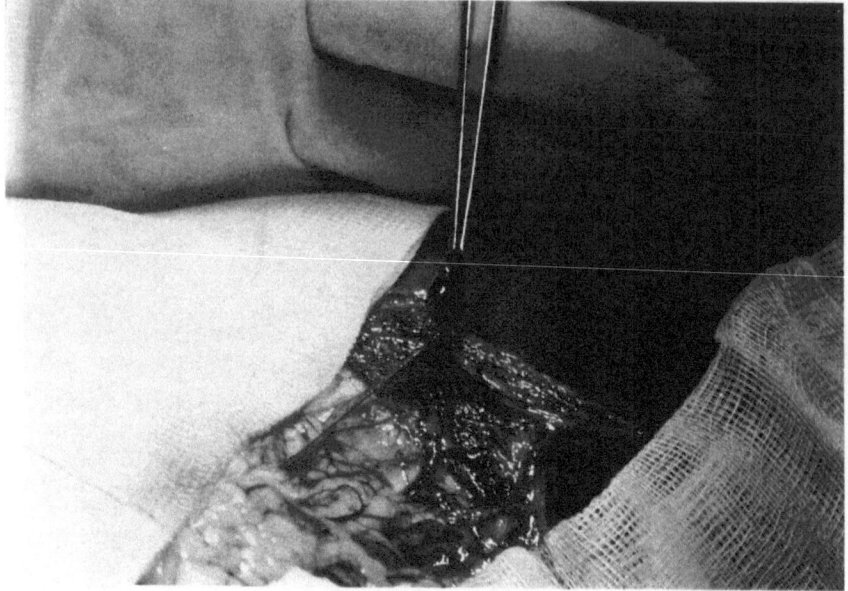

FIGURE 5.3 It is possible to remove the omentum of a child through the 2–3 cm incision necessary for the catheter placement

Care is necessary to align the peritoneum with the required direction of the catheter. The catheter's proximal cuff is pulled through the anterior sheath to make the cuff lie on top and within the rectus muscle (Figure 5.4). A purse string suture holds the cuff in place. The catheter tip is placed caudally in the peritoneal cavity and is checked by a malleable copper introducer. The position of the catheter is assessed and the skin exit site chosen so that the distal cuff is 5–7 cm (Figure 5.5) from the exit and the exit well clear of the nappy line in infants. The spiked introducer is used to make the cephalically directed tunnel and achieve a tight external skin exit. The direction of the catheter within the tunnel and through the sheath is secured with further sutures. The opening of the parietal peritoneum and posterior rectus sheath is closed with a purse string suture. This suture falls underneath the rectus muscle. The anterior rectus sheath is repaired and the wound closed. To protect the catheter from accidental damage by clamps, an extension piece is added.

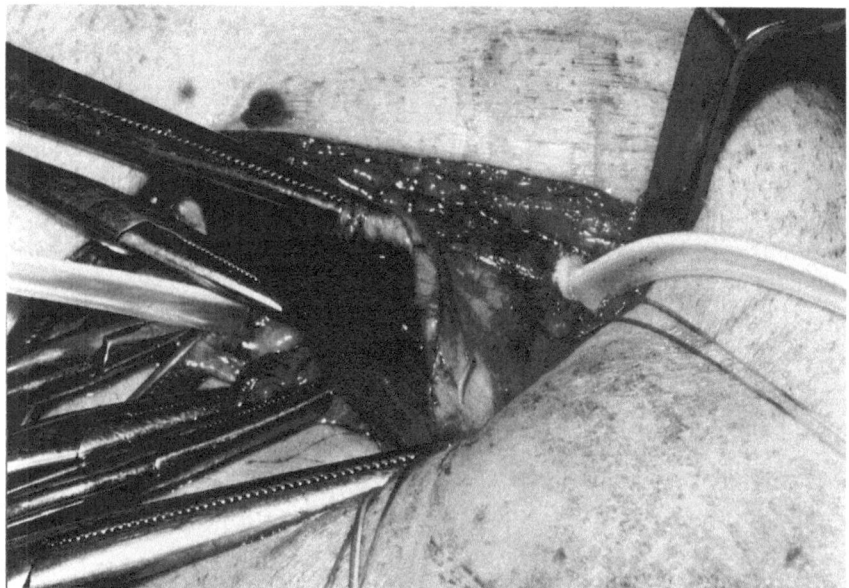

FIGURE 5.4 The double cuff Tenckhoff catheter is inserted through the intact rectus sheath and the proximal cuff is pulled through the anterior sheath to make the cuff lie on top and within the rectus muscle. A purse string suture holds the cuff in place

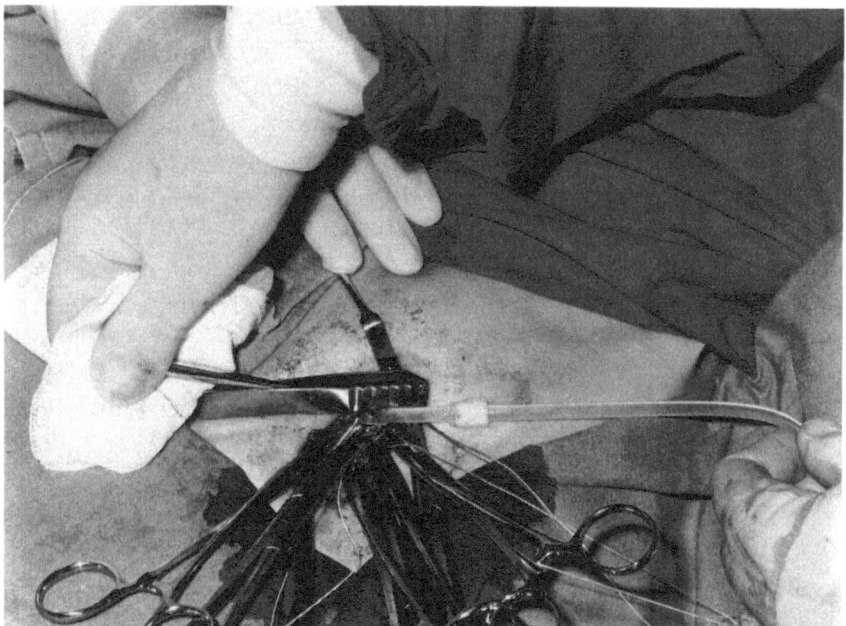

FIGURE 5.5 The catheter tip is placed caudally in the peritoneum. The position of the catheter is assessed and the skin exit site chosen so that the distal cuff is 6–7 cm from the exit

Operative care of exit sites

A retaining suture 6 cm from the skin exit site is always placed around the catheter using prolene. It is left in place for 6–8 weeks and is a reminder not to pull on the catheter, as accidental and careless handling will disturb the cuffs before they can make firm fibrous union with the patient's tissues. This takes at least three months. Unfortunately, reminders and strappings never seem sufficient. A full bag is heavy and can, if accidentally dropped, pull and disturb the healing tunnel. Additional care is achieved by the placing of a corset (Tubepad) or binder, which also supports the abdominal wall and incision. Tube gauze makes an excellent corset and dressing for infants.

Immediate post-operative care

The catheter function is tested in the operating theatre before closure of the wound with volumes of dialysate appropriate to the patient's size, between 30–40 ml/kg body weight. The catheter is also tested immediately post-operatively by performing several exchanges without dwell times over the next two hours. The catheter is then filled with 2 ml of 1000 U/ml heparin and capped off. The catheter is left unused for three weeks to allow wound and tunnel healing. Should the patient have an unexplained temperature or any abdominal discomfort, a check flush is done and the fluid sent for culture. It is important to note that the fluid returned from a check flush of a resting peritoneum is always discoloured and may have more cells than CAPD fluid from an established patient, but the diagnosis of peritonitis is usually straightforward. After each check flush the catheter should be reheparinized.

It is surprising how willingly experienced surgeons will allow physicians to use the catheter immediately, even allowing CAPD within a few days. They would not allow similar soaking and stretching of abdominal wounds in other surgical situations without expecting delayed healing, dehiscence and incisional hernia. Why should they change their technique for a culture medium such as peritoneal dialysis fluid? In centres where peritoneal dialysis is started immediately after catheter insertion, early infection and hernia are reported in 30% of patients[15,18,19].

Dialysis in the post-operative period

If dialysis is essential during the three-week catheter healing period, children larger than 15 kg are electively haemodialysed through a temporary subclavian or femoral vein catheter. For smaller children and infants, short periods of IPD are undertaken with the patient in the recumbent position, and using small volumes sufficient to maintain the biochemistry within acceptable levels. The abdomen needs to be supported with some form of binder or corset and every effort made to ensure that the child is not in distress and crying excessively, otherwise leaking will occur around the catheter and wound resulting in delayed healing, infection, and herniation[13,19]. In the very young, umbilical and inguinal herniae can appear immediately at the first instillation of peritoneal fluid even in patients previously checked for hernia. Leakage into the perineum is common if the catheter is used immediately. It usually reabsorbs if the dialysis is stopped for 48 hours. There is a need to be patient by allowing the peritoneum to adjust to the presence of the dialysate at intervals of 48 hours. If hernias become evident then repair should be planned so that the peritoneum can be rested for several days after operation. This requires extra intensive dialysis prior to operation.

There are some patients where no evidence of hernial weakness can be found but who intermittently at intervals of several months apart will develop swelling into the perineum and or scrotum. There are no related events to cause the leakage which will settle quickly if CAPD is stopped for a few days. If it recurs again within a few days then a programme of twice or thrice weekly IPD for two weeks usually solves the problem.

CAPD DIALYSIS

The standard technique of four exchanges every 24 hours is suitable for children, although for small infants five to six exchanges per day is often necessary. More frequent exchanges are required in small children because there is a more rapid absorption of dialysate dextrose and therefore loss of filtration power of the dialysate than occurs in older children and adults[20]. A volume of 40–50 ml/kg body weight is a guideline for the volume of each exchange. It is wise to start with smaller volumes and then to increase to find the maximum the patient comfortably tolerates. The manufacturers have a range of differently sized bags and strengths, and are also willing to make special-size bags, should the need arise. Changing the composition of the fluid is more difficult to arrange.

Training

Who should do the dialysis

My own personal approach to home dialysis and training differs from others, but it has been derived from 25 years of home haemodialysis and 18 years home peritoneal dialysis experience[21]. The main points are that the dialysis should be the responsibility of only one person; all the teaching should go to that one person until the patient goes home. When the patient is established in the home, the trained person is then at liberty to involve the help of others in the areas in which it is required, provided that the trained individual will take responsibility for the other person or persons and ensure that standards are maintained. By doing this, there is only one method in each household, and arguments and dissention on what 'someone else said' are reduced to a minimum. The various dealings with the family are then usually through one person, which simplifies situations.

Role of children and adolescents

Although the technical side of the treatment is simple and the bag exchanges are made easier by newer equipment, the correct management of a patient with regard to fluid balance, accurate weight and blood pressure recording needs more than being able to do a bag exchange. Children as young as four know every move and the order in which they should be made. Many people believe that children of 12 can take responsibility and perform their own exchanges. They can undertake the exchanges but cannot take the responsibility for the records and fluid adjustments. The twelve-year-old is in many ways safer than the teenage patient as the parents are still in charge. Teenagers, as they get older, want to be completely in charge. They will 'lock out' the parents, not allowing them to check the weights, blood pressure, etc. Unfortunately, this technical ability is rarely matched with the maturity to admit errors in technique or to sustain them with the repetitive drudgery of changing the bag 1500 times a year.

In my own unit, the entire treatment is the responsibility of the parent. No child or teenager is allowed to do an exchange. Children are taught to watch and act as a check on the adult who is doing the treatment. The reasoning for this is explained to the parent and child together. Even the teenagers accept the rules, especially when they realize how boring it becomes.

Choice of system and bag change

There are many new systems and devices to help with the bag exchanges and prevent contamination. None currently in use is free from user error, and the over-riding factor is the ability to recognize an error in technique or equipment and to respond to it immediately by taking preventative action. For example, a dropped line needs immediate change and antibiotic cover. This requires a 24 hour service from the department and an understanding by the family of how to use it. Overall, the bag exchanges are the simplest part of the training and most parents seem to concentrate very well on this aspect and learn quickly.

Blood pressure measurement

There is a need to know the blood pressure in hypertensive children with fluctuating fluid loads. Encouragement is necessary as this often proves the most difficult technical task. The difficulty arises from the background noises and the quietness of the beat in the child who fidgets with the discomfort of the pressure on its arm. The restlessness often precludes the use of the newer equipment where a light responds to the pulse. Mercury sphygmomanometers are often easier to control than pressure spring gauges. The correct cuff size for the patient's arm must be used. It should be two-thirds of the upper arm.

Weight

For small infants and children excellent electronic, relatively inexpensive scales weighing up to 20 kg with either a seat or basket are available. They can be used to weigh the child and, as they measure to the nearest 10 g, are also very accurate for bag weighing to estimate fluid removal. Normal standing, good quality scales are suitable for older children.

Fluid balance and diet

The understanding of fluid balance requires regular daily, followed by weekly, instruction over a period often extending up to three months. This area of training incorporates the diet and fluid intake. It is made significantly more difficult by the feeding problems invariably encountered with children. Infants can defy adult feeding plans by refusing to eat or drink and vomiting regularly after feeding. Children not only do this but add to the frustration by sneaking drinks. This is an area where the child can dictate, and the parents need enormous help to spot the problems and come to terms with the various ways in which the child 'bugs' the system. Parents are frequently indignant if the doctor or nurse suggests the child is taking extra drinks, as their child would never lie. They do not appreciate the extent to which all dialysis patients feel thirsty, especially in the first few months. At this stage, it is necessary to weigh all the bags, both going in and coming out, to see the ultrafiltration achieved and to balance it with the estimated intake and any urine output. The actual regime may need changing daily until a stable state is reached.

The training period in hospital need not be prolonged beyond getting the patient well, but there must be provision for extended

112

teaching at home, by home visits, regular telephone discussions and clinic visits. Parents almost always rise to the demands of the treatment programme regardless of their educational background, and will with patience grasp the skill of fluid balance and nutritional management.

DIETARY REQUIREMENTS

It has been shown by many workers that children in renal failure need at least the minimum recommended dietary allowance for their size or bone age[22-26]. Failure to achieve the recommended intake results in further falls in growth velocity. As these children are usually already below the 50th percentile, with many even below the 3rd, nutrition becomes a vital factor in their management. Catch-up growth is rarely seen until after a successful transplant. With infants accepted for treatment during their first year of life, the aim is to achieve a suitable size for transplantation, usually around 10 kg.

Apart from the calories necessary for growth, allowances have to be made in the diet for protein and essential amino acids lost in the dialysis fluid[27-30]. Fifty percent of the energy should be provided from dietary fat. The ratio of polyunsaturated to saturated fatty acids should be 1.5:1. Some further adjustment of fat intake may be necessary for inherent serum lipid abnormalities[31-35]. The recommended dietary intake for each age group is shown in Table 5.1.

TABLE 5.1   Recommended dietary intake for children on CAPD

Age	Protein (g/kg/day)	Energy (kcal/kg/day)
0–3 years	4–6	110
3–puberty	2.5	Recommended dietary allowance for normal child of same height, bone age
puberty	2	
post puberty	M 1.5	60
	F 1.5	48

Dietary fat 50% of daily energy
Carbohydrate 35% of daily energy
Dialysate 10–12% of daily energy

113

Dietary water, potassium, sodium, calcium and phosphate supplements or restrictions are adjusted according to the biochemistry and the balancing of dialysate, urinary and bowel losses. Constipation can be a serious problem leading to potassium retention and hyperkalaemia; some children, however, may need potassium supplements. Water-soluble vitamins of the B and C group need replacement and regular checking to ensure correct levels. Active vitamin D supplements are necessary. In children, phosphate binders should be calcium rather than aluminium based. The balancing of calcium, phosphate and active vitamin D varies markedly from child to child and, apart from routine biochemistry, monthly parathyroid hormone assays and hand and wrist X-rays are necessary every alternate month.

BIOCHEMICAL CONTROL

The stable biochemical control of patients treated by CAPD should not be compared to haemodialysis with its fluctuating levels. Similarly, serum creatinine levels in infants, children and adults are not comparable as creatinine is related to body muscle mass and is obviously less in children. Variations in urea concentration are dependent on actual protein intake as much as efficiency of dialysis. Thus, the patient must act as his own control for efficiency of dialysis. Comparisons of dialysate taken from the overnight bag, usually an 8 hour dwell, and the serum biochemistry measurements of urea, creatinine, sodium, and potassium will indicate the efficiency of the peritoneal membrane. At 8 hours the results are almost identical. Repeat measurements at two-monthly intervals are valuable indications of membrane function. Low urea measurements in children should be regarded suspiciously as a failure to eat sufficient protein rather than simple good biochemical control[36]. Calcium movement into or out of the patient varies greatly from patient to patient. In the early days of peritoneal dialysis children may have raised serum calcium concentration until their vitamin D supplements are adjusted. Serum phosphate concentration is better controlled than in haemodialysis in spite of the higher protein intake. Acidosis is corrected in CAPD and maintained stable unlike the swings seen in haemodialysis[37,38].

Following attention to ensure adequate iron stores and folate and

B_{12} levels, haemoglobin levels will rise initially with the improvement of the uraemic state. They never reach the levels seen in the adult CAPD patients. Like adults, however, transfusion requirements are less than for haemodialysis patients. Falls in haemoglobin are in my experience seen at about a year and reflect some loss of peritoneal function shown by the serum/dialysate differential. The anaemia is tolerated well by most patients but appetites improve with higher haemoglobin concentrations. Early reports[32,38], noted low serum albumin levels in both adults and children but with improvements in techniques and reduction in peritonitis rates, the albumin levels seen today in all groups of patients are well within the normal range. During an episode of peritonitis the serum albumin will fall rapidly but will respond to increased protein intake as soon as the patient can eat normally again. The loss of immunoglobulins into the dialysate may in theory cause IgG deficiency and could lead to increased infections in children. This has not been my experience as children have fewer episodes of peritonitis than adults. In order to overcome the losses of amino acids from the dialysate, fluids with amino acids instead of glucose have been tried, at intervals, over the years. The amino acid is successful in ultrafiltration but it seems the value does not warrant the expense of its production. In the situation of a 'failure to thrive child' amino acids can be added to normal dialysate more economically.

FEEDING

Dietary requirements have been discussed but are difficult to achieve in practice. Anorexia is a major component of renal failure in infants and children. Unlike most adults, it remains a major problem in almost all children, even after improvement in the uraemic state. Infants, as stated previously, may refuse the breast and bottle or take most of the day to ingest a third of the necessary feed. Seventy percent of the dialysate glucose is absorbed[40], and it is suggested that these calories and the presence of the fluid in the abdomen are the cause of the anorexia. This is not the full explanation as children who are haemodialysed are also anorexic. After a reasonable time of natural feeding without success, nasogastric tube feeding may be necessary. Vomiting after each feed may occur. This is dealt with by reducing the volume and giving small volumes more often or by slow infusion overnight. Some children may have the tube inserted nightly by the parents or fine soft silk catheters can be left *in situ* for months. Children soon learn to tolerate the tube and will stop pulling it out if it is always replaced immediately. Patients with persistent vomiting may need transpyloric feeding[41,42]. Others report the use of gastrotomies[43] or parenteral feeding.

Tube feeding may seem to be an acceptance of failure but the time and effort involved in feeding these children exhausts all energies and endangers the other nursing and medical needs of the child. All semblance of family survival is at risk. If the infant does not obtain the calories there will be no growth to the size necessary for transplantation and the whole treatment programme fails. There are several advantages of tube feeding. The feed can be accurately prescribed and mixed, and all the necessary vitamins, minerals and drugs added without the child having to taste unpleasant flavours or textures. Often it is the texture of the food which puts the child off eating. The feed is mixed once a day and kept in the fridge. It is the normal practice to continue breast or bottle feeding in infants but not to consider it the main source of calories. Children are also encouraged to eat freely when being tube fed.

Eating skills may not be acquired by anorexic small children. This must be considered when advising parents about diets and eating expectation. The need for tube feeding may have to be considered at any age. When a child eats normally the diet in CAPD is easy to apply. The main restriction is salty foods, as this increases their existing thirst. Other foods which have high water content should be limited. A good mixed diet of fresh home-cooked foods can be freely served to the child and family together, without fear of problems.

Growth

Linear growth is the most sensitive indicator of health in persons with growth potential. Stress can temporarily affect growth. Enthusiasm for growth potential in CAPD was high as the stable and more normal biochemistry achieved by CAPD and the untraumatic delivery of the treatment in the patient's home augured well. Simple measurement of height at out-patients visits are only a guideline, as they are notoriously inaccurate. It is necessary to have experts take regular measurements. Unfortunately, they have shown that although growth occurred, it is between 70% and 100% of expected height velocity; some patients grew less than 70% of expected height velocity and therefore had severe growth failure[35-38,44,45]. However, children on CAPD are growing better than the historical controls treated by haemodialysis[8,23,46,47]. Children less than two years old and on CAPD grow much better than those maintained by conservative management and thus have a better future height potential[14]. Their ability to grow sufficiently to enable transplantation to be undertaken opens a new perspective in the treatment of ESRF.

RENAL OSTEODYSTROPHY

The problems of renal osteodystrophy (ROD) in children require much more acute management than is necessary in the fully grown adult. Bone turnover is much greater and the development of osteitis fibrosa is very rapidly seen in its most florid forms. High levels of PTH are associated with a decrease in growth velocity[36]. Monthly measurements of PTH are essential to assess control. X-rays of the hand and wrist every two months are also necessary. Skilled adjustment of active vitamin D metabolites and calcium supplements can control both phosphate levels and the parathyroid gland activity, although PTH levels will always be above normal. Parathyroidectomy in children is relatively rarely required as most can be transplanted before this is necessary. In general, the dose of vitamin D necessary to control PTH is high and reflects the loss of vitamin D metabolites in the dialysate.

PERITONITIS

Peritonitis can be devastating in small children. It must be treated by experts and not at the local hospital, however convenient a solution that may appear at the time. The need for accurate microbiology requires temporary hospital admission until the organism is identified and the correct antibiotic has taken effect. Thereafter the treatment can be continued at home. The management is the same as that for adults – cultures of peritoneal fluid in blood culture media and direct plates, and microscopy of the fluid. Blood cultures are necessary especially if the child has a temperature. Swabbing of exit sites, perineum and nose are routine, but there is reward in also swabbing the mouth as it is a frequent source of unusual infections. Children suck and bite anything to hand and will push their fingers into holes unrecognized by adults!

Some microbiologists and paediatricians are reluctant to use ototoxic antibiotics but the best management currently is a combination of vancomycin and an aminoglycoside. This therapy is more specific than a broad spectrum antibiotic such as a cephalosporin, which leaves the patient open to secondary fungal infections that obliterate the peritoneal cavity. In small infants automatic transfer to haemodialysis may not be possible. Newer less toxic antibiotics such as teicoplanin and aztreonam are currently being evaluated and it is hoped that these will be as effective. Whichever antibiotic is chosen, the dosage must be adjusted by regular blood levels as the response to dosage not only varies from child to child but from day to day. During a severe episode of peritonitis the loss of protein and amino acids into the dialysate is very high. The child may vomit or have complete ileus and will certainly have no appetite. Parenteral feeding may be necessary with addition of amino acids to the dialysate.

During episodes of peritonitis, serum amylase is often minimally raised and occasionally significantly raised; the levels return to normal as the peritonitis resolves. Rising levels should be a cause of concern; when this occurs in conjunction with CAPD peritonitis, the best management is the removal of the catheter, although peritoneal lavage has frequently been suggested as the primary treatment of pancreatitis (personal observations).

PREVENTION OF INFECTIONS AND OTHER SUCH PROBLEMS

The need for nappies due to the incontinence of infants increases the risks of infection of the exit site and connections (Figure 5.6). In principle, the surgeon should have ensured that the exit site is well above

118

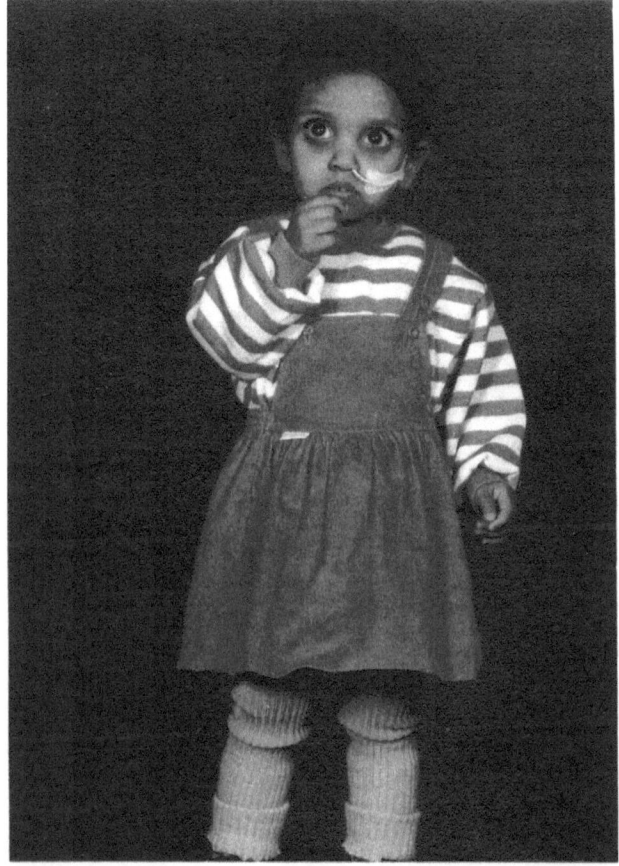

(a)

FIGURE 5.6 This series of photographs of a 22-month-old girl illustrates the problems encountered in small children (a) She came to the UK four months before the photographs were taken, having developed renal failure four months earlier. CAPD was started in her own country where the first catheter needed replacement after 3 months. She had also experienced two severe episodes of peritonitis. On arrival she had evidence of malnutrition with dry skin and no hair. Although she was socially aware of eating, always trying to feed others, she would not eat or drink herself. Thus the need for the nasogastric tube. She continued nasogastric feeding for six months whilst awaiting transplantation. (b) The photograph of her abdomen shows the catheter to be too low and not free of the nappy area. It should have exited level with the taping. There is also a small umbilical hernia. The catheter is taped to her upper abdomen and both the catheter and the hernia are held firm by the Netelast dressing. The connection between the catheter and the line is by her shoulder. The connection is wrapped in a Betadine soaked gauze and firmly taped. (c) The empty dialysate bag and line are folded and slipped into the bag worn on her back. When dressed she is unable to interfere or damage her bag system and is free to play as a normal child

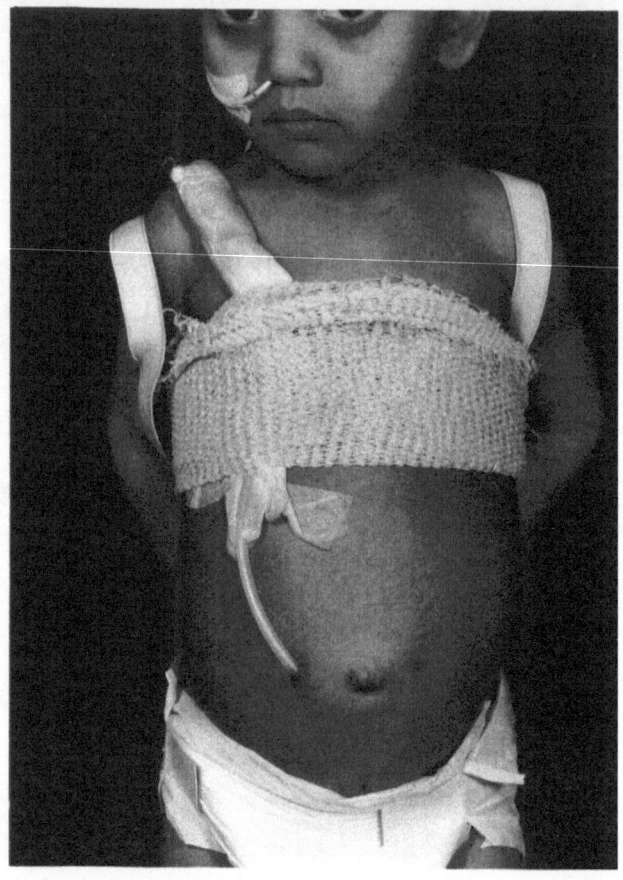

(b)

the nappy line. In the anuric child with regular well-formed stools and regular bowel action, the parent can easily cope with the problem. The wet child with diarrhoea is always at risk. The normal care is to bath the child in Betadine scrub daily and clean the exit area regularly with Betadine. A dry dressing to the exit site is recommended – if it is found to be wet at any time it must be assumed to be contaminated and in need of changing. Similar management points apply to the older child with ureterostomy or ileal conduit. It is important to cover all connections with dry dressings which cannot be disturbed or destroyed as young children will try to pull them apart or chew them. The catheter and bag must be aligned not to interfere with the child's activities. The line, if brought straight up the chest wall and over the

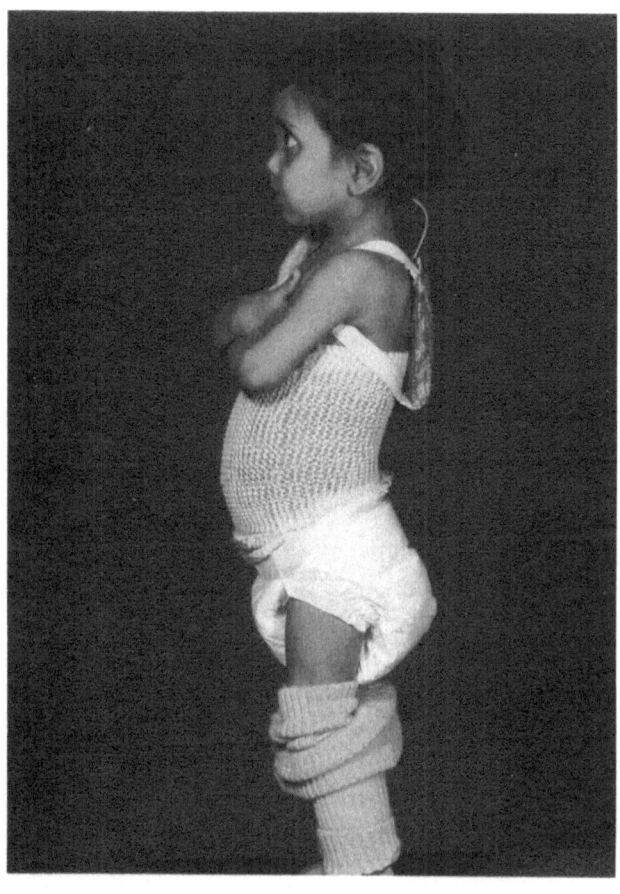

(c)

shoulder, enables the bag to be put in a small backpack. When clothes are worn it is impossible for the child to get at the system and the child becomes unaware of its presence. It is my experience that parents, given advice and practical ideas, will find efficient ways of handling their child. There are some parents who have no insight into their child's activities and in these situations accidents occur. Equipment may get broken or contaminated and a lot can be achieved with a pair of scissors in small hands! Most situations can be retrieved if the parents are not too embarrassed or unconcerned to bring the child to the hospital at once. It is in these situations that prophylactic antibiotics are needed to prevent the almost inevitable peritonitis seen after breaks in technique.

121

SUPPORT SERVICES

Compared to the adult dialysis population, there are not many children being dialysed. Treatment on the whole is successful for the child but the strain on the family is enormous. When things go wrong the threat to life is greater and the options fewer than for adults. A centre planning a children's programme should ensure a higher staff/patient ratio to provide home tuition and support within the home. It is only in the patient's home that you can assess general hygiene, quality of diet and family eating habits. Social reports from outside persons are of limited value when providing total medical care. The doctor's role is directed to assessing medical progress and ensuring the quality of the techniques used. Visits to the home by trained CAPD nursing staff are greatly appreciated. Training and skills acquired in the hospital setting need to be translated for each particular home. It is frequently necessary to discuss methods of dealing with the other children's demands in such a way that they do not feel jealous and distract the parent during vital treatment times. The trained staff can help plan the arrangement of the equipment and stores. They also need to show parents how to turn over and order their stock. The home CAPD nurse should pay regular visits to the home for reinforcement of techniques and introduction of new ideas. Frequently, new ideas are rejected at first but if worked out in the home prove to be welcome. The CAPD nurse is the one person most likely to discover the recurrent technical errors or the tricks the child might be up to which are causing the medical problems. When children return to school the home nurse assesses the feasibility of bag exchanges by the mother at school – most schools have medical rooms. This requires that the home CAPD nurse and the parent meet the teachers and the school nurse. The school nurse may offer to perform the exchanges but this offer should be declined, as the commitment to the child and technical skills are never as great as the parent. There is always a reluctance to accept the child back at school as the staff are frightened that some accident will occur. The CAPD nurse can assure them of the simplicity of the treatment and the need to treat the child as normal. When exchanges cannot be undertaken at school or the parent cannot give the time in the middle of the day then the exchanges may be reduced to three on school days with four at the weekends. All varieties of bag exchange programmes may be necessary to fit in with family commitments. It is important to get the family to combine flexibility with discipline in their treatment regime, otherwise parents become obsessed with doing exchanges exactly on the hour regardless of other commitments. Needless to say the child's life becomes severely restricted too.

The dietician plays a vital role in the progress of a child on CAPD. Theirs is a difficult task requiring regular assessments of dietary intake, without adding extra stress to the parents. My own observations are that pressure to get the calories into the child results in the child remaining the same and the parent getting fatter!

THE ROLE OF IPD/CCPD IN THE MANAGEMENT OF CHILDREN

CAPD gives better biochemical control than the other forms of peritoneal dialysis. There are, however, several situations where intermittent resting of the peritoneum is medically valuable. Without doubt episodes of peritonitis are reduced[48]. It seems that the scavenging properties of the white cells of the peritoneum are improved after a period of rest even a few hours each day. When lost, ultrafiltration may return after complete or intermittent rest. My own experience of CCPD over 18 years has shown that the peritoneum functions for up to nine years, whereas in CAPD it is limited to six years. No one is expecting children to remain on dialysis for long periods so the above problems should not have to be seriously considered. The problem of infection is certainly important and where a patient is having mild recurrent episodes of peritonitis a change to CCPD may well solve the problem. The reduction in infection rate may also be due to the need for only one sterile procedure daily.

Most of the reasons for undertaking CCPD in favour if CAPD relate to the convenience of schooling or parents' work patterns. Some children prefer having no peritoneal fluid all day and for some children there may be an improvement in appetite when their abdomen is no longer distended.

CONCLUSION

CAPD is an excellent form of treatment for end-stage renal failure in infants and children. It is of particular importance in those under two years old – it is now implemented in patients previously managed by conservative therapy in order to ensure growth during the vital period.

Success in CAPD is dependent on meticulous attention to detail, especially in the tuition of the caring parent. Good placement and healing of the peritoneal catheter is more difficult than in adults because of the diminished area and lack of depth of the abdominal wall necessary for successful tunnelling.

In those centres which have mastered the techniques of CAPD it is now used extensively for young patients. The reduced transfusion requirements during CAPD treatment minimizes the risk of trans-fusion-acquired antibodies. Although biochemistry is not so well controlled, and the treatment is more expensive, there is a tendency to use more CCPD in children as it is often more convenient for the family.

REFERENCES

1. Drukker, W., Haagsma-Schouten, W. A. G., Alberts, Chr., & Spoek, M. G. (1969). Report on regular dialysis treatment in Europe, V, 1969. *Proc. Eur. Dial. Transplant Assoc.*, **6**, 99–108
2. Levin, S., Winklestein, J. A. (1967). Diet and infrequent peritoneal dialysis in chronic anuric uremia. *N. Engl. J. Med.*, **277**, 619
3. Donckerwolcke, R. A., Chantler, C., Broyer, M. *et al.* (1979). Combined report on regular dialysis and transplantation of children in Europe. *Proc. Eur. Dial. Transplant Assoc.*, **17**, 89
4. Popovich, R. P., Moncrief, J. W., Decherd, J. F. *et al.* (1976). The definition of a novel portable, wearable equilibrium peritoneal dialysis technique. *Am. Soc. Artif. Intern. Organs*, **5**, 64A (abstract)
5. Alexander, S. R., Tseng, C. H., Maksym, K. A. *et al.* (1980). Early clinical experience with continuous ambulatory peritoneal dialysis (CAPD) in infants and children. *Clin. Res.*, **128**, 131A
6. Balfe, J. W., Vigneux, A., Willumsen, J. *et al.* (1981). The use of CAPD in the treatment of children with end stage renal disease. *Perit. Dial. Bull.*, **1**, 35
7. Popovich, R. P., Moncrief, J. W., Nolph, K. D., *et al.* (1978). Continuous ambulatory peritoneal dialysis. *Ann. Intern. Med.*, **88**, 449
8. Broyer, M., Rizzoni, G., Brunner, F-P., Brynger, H., Challah, S., Fassbinder, W., Oules, R., Selwood, N. H. and Wing, A. J. (1985). Combined report on

regular dialysis and transplantation of children in Europe XIV, 1984. *Proc. Eur. Dial. Transplant Assoc. ERA*, **22**, 55–78

9. Betts, P. R., McGrath, G. (1972). Growth pattern and dietary intake in children with chronic renal insufficiency. *Br. Med. J.*, **2**, 189

10. Rotundo, A., Nevins, T. E., Lipton, M. *et al.* (1982). Progressive encephalopathy in children with chronic renal insufficiency in infancy. *Kidney Int.*, **21**, 486

11. Baluarte, J. H., Gruskin, A. B., Hiner, L. B. *et al.* (1977). Encephalopathy in children with chronic renal failure. *Proc. Dial. Transplant Forum*, **7**, 95

12. Geary, D. F., Fennell, R. S., Andriola, M. *et al.* (1983). Encephalopathy in children with chronic renal failure. *J. Pediat.*, **96**, 41

13. Fonkalsrud, E. W. (1987). Peritoneal catheter; technique, longevity, complications. In Fine RN (ed) *Chronic Ambulatory Peritoneal Dialysis (CAPD) and Chronic Cycling Peritoneal Dialysis (CCPD) in Children*, pp. 111–122. (Boston/Dordrecht: Martinus Nijhoff)

14. Kohaut, E. C. (1987). CAPD in infants. In Fine RN (ed) *Chronic Ambulatory Peritoneal Dialysis (CAPD) and Chronic Cycling Peritoneal Dialysis (CCPD) in Children*, pp. 77–86. (Boston/Dordrecht: Martinus Nijhoff)

15. Orkin, B. A., Fonkalsrud, E. W., Salusky, I. B. *et al.* (1983). Continuous ambulatory peritoneal dialysis catheters in children. *Arch. Surg.*, **118**, 1398

16. Helfrich, G. B., Pechan, B. W., Alijani, M. R. *et al.* (1983). Reduction of catheter complications with lateral placement. *Perit. Dial. Bull.* (Suppl), **3**, S2

17. Baillod, R. A. (1988). A new surgical approach to peritoneal catheter placement technique. *Perit. Dial. Int. VIII Annual CAPD, Abstracts,* 7

18. Swartz, R. D. (1985). Chronic peritoneal dialysis; mechanical and infectious complications. *Nephron*, **40**, 29

19. Watson, A. R., Vigneux, A., Hardy, B. E., Balfe, J. W. (1985). Six years experience with CAPD catheters in children. *Perit. Dial. Bull*, **5**, 119

20. Kohaut, E. C., Alexander, S. (1981). Ultrafiltration in the young patient on CAPD. In Moncrief, J. W., Popovich, R. P. (eds) *CAPD Update*, p. 221. (New York:Masson)

21. Baillod, R. A. (1983). Home dialysis. In Drukker, W., Parsons, F. M., Maher, J. F. (eds) *Replacement of Renal Function by Dialysis*, pp. 493–513. (Boston/Dordrecht:Martinus Nijhoff)

22. Simmons, J. M., Wilson, C. J., Potter D. E. *et al.* (1971). Relation of calorie deficiency to growth failure in children on haemodialysis and the growth response to calorie supplementation. *N. Engl. J. Med.*, **285**, 653

23. Kleinknecht, C., Broyer, M., Gagnadoux, M. F. *et al.* (1980). Growth in children treated with long term dialysis. In Hamburger, J., Crosmier, J., Grunfield, J. P. (eds) *Advances in Nephrology*, **9**, 133

24. Rizzoni, G., Basso, T., Setari, M. (1984). Growth in children with chronic renal failure on conservative treatment. *Kidney Int.*, **26**, 52

25. Chantler, C., El-Bishti, M., Counahan, R. (1980). Nutritional therapy in children with chronic renal failure. *Am. J. Clin. Nutr.*, **33**, 1682

26. Wassner, S. J., Abitbol, C., Alexander, S. *et al.* (1986). Nutrition and dialysis requirements for infants with renal failure. *Am. J. Kidney Dis.*, **7**, 300

27. Dulaney, J. T., Hatch, F. E. (1984). Peritoneal dialysis and loss of protein: a review. *Kidney Int.*, **26**, 253

28. Giordano, C., De Santo, N. G., Pluvio, M. *et al.* (1980). Protein requirement of patients on CAPD: a study on nitrogen balance. *Int. J. Artif. Organs*, **3**, 11

29. Blumenkrantz, M. J., Gahl, G. M., Kopple, J. D. *et al.* (1981). Protein losses during peritoneal dialysis. *Kidney Int.*, **19**, 593
30. Giordano, C., De Santo, N. G., Capodicesa, G. (1981). Amino acid losses during CAPD in children. *Int. J. Pediat. Nephrol.*, **2**, 85
31. Sanfelippo, M. L., Swenson, R. S., Reaven, G. M. (1977). Reduction of plasma triglycerides by diet in subjects with chronic renal failure. *Kidney Int.*, **11**, 54
32. Chan, M. K., Chuah, P., Raftery, M. J. *et al.* (1981). Three years' experience of continuous ambulatory dialysis. *Lancet*, **1**, 1409
33. Lindhold, B., Bergstrom, J., Norbeck, H. E. (1981). Lipoprotein metabolism in patients on continuous ambulatory peritoneal dialysis. In Gahl, G. M., Kessel, M., Nolph, K. D. (eds) *Advances in Peritoneal Dialysis*, p. 434. (Amsterdam:Excerpta Medica)
34. Pennisi, A. J., Henser, E. T., Mickey, M. R. *et al.* (1976). Hyperlipidemia in pediatric haemodialysis and renal transplant patients. *Am. J. Dis. Child.*, **130**, 957
35. Salusky, I. B., Fine, R. N., Nelson, P. *et al.* (1983). Nutritional status of children undergoing continuous ambulatory peritoneal dialysis. *Am. J. Clin. Nutr.*, **38**, 599
36. Kohaut, E. C., Waldo, F. B. (1987). Growth in children on CAPD. In Fine, R. N. (ed) *Chronic Ambulatory Peritoneal Dialysis (CAPD) and Chronic Cycling Peritoneal Dialysis (CCPD) in Children*, pp. 289–296. (Boston:Martinus Nijhoff)
37. Baum, M., Powell, D., Calvin, J. (1982). Continuous ambulatory peritoneal dialysis in children: comparison with haemodialysis. *N. Engl. J. Med.*, **307**, 1537
38. Kohaut, E. C. (1983). Growth in children treated with continuous ambulatory peritoneal dialysis. *Int. J. Pediat. Nephrol.*, **4**, 93
39. Broyer, M., Niaudet, P., Champion, G. *et al.* (1983). Nutrition and metabolic studies in children on continuous ambulatory peritoneal dialysis. *Kidney Int.*, **24**, S16
40. Kopple, J. D., Blumenkrantz, M. J. (1983). Nutritional requirements for patients undergoing continuous ambulatory peritoneal dialysis. *Kidney Int.*, **24**, S16
41. Conley, S. B., Brewer, E. D., Grady, S. *et al.* (1982). Normal growth in very small children on peritoneal dialysis. Program and Abstracts, National Kidney Foundation, December 3–13, 1982, Chicago, IL, 8
42. Brewer, E. D., Holmes, S., Tealey, J. (1985). Initiation and maintenance of growth in infants with ESRD managed with CAPD and nasogastric feeding. Abstracts, American Society of Nephrology, December 15–18, 1985, New Orleans, LA, p. 81A
43. O'Regan, S., Garel, L. (1988). Percutaneous gastrojejunostomy for tube feeding in children with end-stage renal disease. *Perit. Dial. Int, VIII Annual CAPD Abstracts*, 120
44. Stefanidis, C. J., Hewitt, I. K., Balfe, J. W. (1983). Growth in children receiving continuous ambulatory peritoneal dialysis. *J. Pediat.*, **102**, 681
45. Fennell, R. S., Orak, J. K., Hudson, T. *et al.* (1984). Growth in children with various therapies for end-stage renal disease. *Am. J. Dis. Child.*, **138**, 28
46. Chantler, C., Carter, J. E., Bewick, M., *et al.* (1980). Ten years experience with haemodialysis in renal transplants. *Am. Dis. Child.*, **55**, 435
47. Mehls, O., Ritz, E. Gilli, G. *et al.* (1978). Growth in renal failure. *Nephron*, **21**, 237
48. Baillod, R. A. (1980). Continuous ambulatory peritoneal dialysis versus intermittent peritoneal dialysis at the Royal Free Hospital. In Legrain M. (ed) *Continuous Ambulatory Peritoneal Dialysis*, p. 328. (Amsterdam:Excerpta Medica)

INDEX

albumin 16, 17
aldosterone 13
Alkaligenes spp. 40
aluminium toxicity 14
amino acids 7
  metabolism 16–17
  muscle free 17
anaemia 12
anaerobic bacteria 40, 42
asparagine 17
aspartic acid 17

Bacillus spp. 40
bacteraemia 19

C3 21
calcium 13–14
calcium carbonate 14
calcium channel antagonists 25
Canadian Renal Failure Registry 26
Candida spp. 39–40
carbohydrate metabolism 15
cardiomyopathies 59
catheters 9–11
  break-in technique 10 (table)
  colonization 20–1
  complications 10 (table)
  fluid leak 10 (table)
  insertion 10 (table)
  material 10 (table)
  obstruction 10 (table)
cell-mediated immune function 22 (fig)
children, CAPD in 99–124
  anaemia 114–15
  anorexia 115
  biochemical control 114–15
  blood pressure measurement 111
  dialysis 109–111
    bag change 111
    choice of system 111

    post-operative period 109
    role of children/adolescents 110
  diet 112–14
  dietician 123
  feeding 115–16
  fluid balance 112–13
  growth 116–17
  haemoglobin 115
  home CAPD nurse 122–3
  immunoglobin loss 115
  infants 101
  infection prevention 118
  peritonitis 100–1, 117–18
  postoperative care 108–9
  renal osteodystrophy 117
  support services 122–3
  technique 102–13
    anaesthetic 103
    catheter choice/insertion 103
    incision 104
    omentum examination 104
    operation 105–7
    operative care of exit sites 108
  unsuitable patients 100–1
  vomiting 115–16
  weight 112
  when to start 101–2
Citrobacter spp. 40
citrulline 17
'colloid' osmosis 8
continuous ambulatory peritoneal
  dialysis (CAPD)
  adequacy 17–18
  advantages/disadvantages 11 (table)
  children *see* children
  clinical results 11
  diabetes patients *see* diabetes mellitus
  elderly patient *see* elderly patient
  equipment 8–11
    catheters *see* catheters

127